Handbook of Pediatric Orthopedics

Handbook of Pediatric Orthopedics

Paul D. Sponseller, M.D.

Associate Professor, Department of Orthopedic Surgery
Johns Hopkins University School of Medicine
Director, Division of Pediatric Orthopedics
Johns Hopkins Hospital, Baltimore

Heidi M. Stephens, M.D.

Assistant Professor, Department of Orthopedic Surgery
University of South Florida College of Medicine, Tampa

Little, Brown and Company

Boston   New York   Toronto   London

Library of Congress Cataloging-in-Publication Data

Sponseller, Paul D.
    Handbook of pediatric orthopedics / Paul D. Sponseller and Heidi M. Stephens.
        p.   cm.
    Includes bibliographical references and index.
    ISBN 0-316-80872-5
    1. Pediatric orthopedics--Handbooks, manuals, etc.   I. Title.
    [DNLM: 1. Orthopedics--in infancy & childhood--handbooks.   WS 39
    S763h 1996]
    RD732.3.C48S66   1996
    617.3'0083--dc20
    DNLM/DLC
for Library of Congress   96-6386
                                                 CIP

Printed in the United States of America
RRD-VA

Editorial: Nancy E. Chorpenning, Michelle LaPlante
Production Services: Silverchair Science + Communications
Copyeditor: Joan Kocsis
Production Supervisor/Cover Designer: Mike Burggren
Cover drawing by Livia Sponseller, age 6.

Contents

Preface

The *Handbook of Pediatric Orthopedics* will be a useful reference in the care of children with musculoskeletal problems.

There are several excellent texts that describe the theory and practice of children's orthopedics. From these, one may gain concepts and an understanding of pathology. However, many times specific information is needed to diagnose a problem to interpret a radiograph or test, or to plan treatment. The purpose of this text is to provide factual information and guidelines that cannot always be carried around in one's head.

The first chapter provides guidelines on normal growth and development. Normal radiographic values are included, as well as a description of normal gait. The second chapter summarizes selected pediatric orthopedic conditions. The third chapter outlines the treatment of skeletal trauma. Fourth is an outline of syndrome and heritable disorders we commonly encounter, in case there isn't time to consult the literature. These are grouped by presenting features, such as short stature, marfanoid habitus, extremity malformation, and so forth. The fifth chapter describes trauma of the spinal cord and peripheral nerves. The sixth chapter contains a description of techniques such as arthrograms, aspiration, nerve blocks, and traction, which fall mainly within the province of children's orthopedics. Finally, the appendix provides normal laboratory values and dosages and information on medication commonly used in our subspecialty.

Critical to this book was the dedicated help of Jane Kier-York, RN, and Sue Martin, PA, and advice from J. David Thompson, MD. We appreciate the encouragement of our editor, Nancy Chorpenning, and the thoroughness of Elizabeth Willingham. We dedicate this to all of our residents, who taught us as we taught them.

P.D.S.
H.M.S.

Handbook of
Pediatric
Orthopedics

Notice

The indications and dosages of all drugs in this book have been recommended in the medical literature and conform to the practices of the general medical community. The medications described do not necessarily have specific approval by the Food and Drug Administration for use in the diseases and dosages for which they are recommended. The package insert for each drug should be consulted for use and dosage as approved by the FDA. Because standards for usage change, it is advisable to keep abreast of revised recommendations, particularly those concerning new drugs.

Normal Development and Anatomy

Knowledge of normal growth and development is important for evaluation of both the normal and the neurologically or physically abnormal child. This chapter presents anatomic and developmental norms for the skeleton and relevant areas of the nervous system. The normal gait is described, and guidelines are given for interpreting a gait study.

Chapter Outline

I. Neurodevelopmental norms. When evaluating a patient with a risk of developmental delay, the physician needs to know normal developmental values to determine whether or not a delay is present. Appropriate assistance may then be sought. Section A of this chapter presents the typical chronologic appearance of certain key motor, social, and language skills. The Denver Developmental Screening II test (Fig. 1-1) gives the same information in an expanded, graphic form. The Denver II is a graphic representation of developmental norms gathered from 1969 to 1990 from more than 2,000 children from birth to age 6. Norms are also available for various ethnic groups, which is important because some motor norms differ for African-American children. Although the orthopedic surgeon does not perform the test, it provides an excellent summary of developmental milestones for reference. The Denver II forms and manual contain the ethnic norms as well as the test kit. These can be obtained from:

Denver Developmental Materials, Inc.
P.O. Box 6919
Denver, Colorado 80206-0919
(800) 419-4729

A. Psychomotor skills in children during years 1–5*

Neonatal period (first month):
Supine:	Generally flexed and tone a little stiff

2 months:
Prone:	Head sustained in plane of body in ventral suspension
Social:	Smiles on social contact

4 months:
Supine:	Reaches and grasps objects and brings them to mouth
Sitting:	No head lag on pull to sitting position

4–6 months:
Semantics:	Turns to his or her name

7 months:
Prone:	Rolls over
Sitting:	Sits briefly, with support of pelvis
Adaptive:	Transfers objects from hand to hand

10 months:
Standing:	Pulls to standing position
Motor:	Creeps or crawls

12–18 months:
Syntax:	Speech generally consists of single-word utterances (comment)

12 months:
Motor:	Walks with one hand held, "cruises" or walks holding on to furniture
Language:	2 "words" besides mama, dada

15 months:
Motor:	Walks alone, crawls up stairs

---

* Source: Behrman (ed). *Nelson Textbook of Pediatrics* (14th ed). Philadelphia: Saunders, 1992. Pp 41–46.

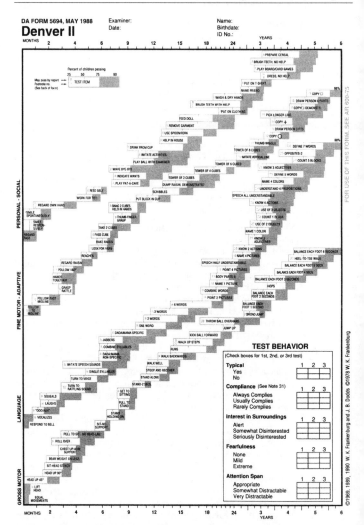

Fig. 1-1. Denver Developmental Screening Test II. (Reproduced with permission from W Frankenburg, J Dodds, P Archer et al. The Denver II: A major revision and restandardization of the Denver Developmental Screening Test. *Pediatrics* 89:91, 1992.)

18 months:
    Motor: Runs stiffly
    Social: Feeds self
24 months:
    Motor: Opens doors
    Syntax: Uses two- and three-word combinations (telegraphic speech)
30 months:
    Motor: Jumps
36 months
    Motor: Goes up stairs alternating feet, stands momentarily on one foot
48 months:
    Motor: Hops on one foot, throws ball overhand
60 months:
    Motor: Skips

B. Referral should be made if the child is
1. Not rolling by **6 months**
2. Not sitting independently by **8 months**
3. Handedness develops too early (by **12 months**): may indicate abnormality of opposite side
4. Not walking by **18 months**
5. No words by **14 months**

C. The **Denver II test** (see Fig. 1-1)
1. This test can be used on children from **birth to age 6.** It is used to determine which children must be referred for diagnostic evaluation. It is not an IQ test. The Denver II test has four sections: personal-social, fine motor, language, and gross motor. Although the orthopedic surgeon does not administer the test, the chart provides an excellent summary of motor development.
2. **Instructions.** Make the child comfortable. He or she may sit on the parent's lap. Correct for prematurity if relevant. Draw a vertical line through the age. Test all intersected boxes and at least three items to the left of it. The child may have three trials to perform each before scoring a failure.
3. **Scoring.** P = pass; F = fail; N.O. = no opportunity; C = caution: child fails or refuses an item that 75–90% of children perform correctly; D = delay: child failed item to left of age line completely; Abnormal = 2 or more delays: refer for diagnostic evaluation. If the child is unable to perform any item, administer items to the left until the child passes 3 items.

II. Neurologic anatomy
A. Sensation. Knowledge of **dermatomes** (Fig. 1-2) is helpful in the evaluation of neurologic conditions. There is, however, some variation and overlap between segmental levels. Injury to a single nerve root may not produce complete loss of sensation within a dermatome. Sensation should be recorded as increased, decreased, absent, or dysesthetic. The sensation of proprioception and vibration is carried in the dorsal column, light touch in the ventral spinothalamic tract, and pain and temperature in the lat-

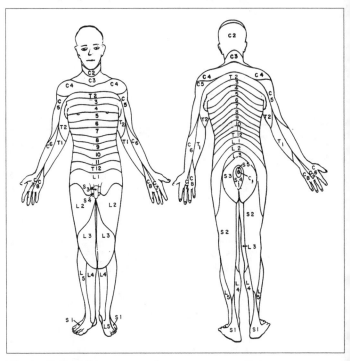

Fig. 1-2. Dermatomes.

eral spinothalamic tract. During neurologic root recovery, pain sensation returns before light touch.

B. Upper extremity motor examination. Injury to the roots or the cord of the cervical spine follows certain patterns. Even though most muscles have innervation from multiple spinal segments, each root has specific muscles and sensory regions for which it is critical. The illustrations in Figure 1-3 are helpful for diagnosing cervical root lesions and spinal cord injury. Motor testing can be performed in one coordinated sequence, from proximal to distal: deltoid (C5), biceps (C5), wrist extension (C6), finger extension (C7), finger flexion (C8), and finger abduction and adduction (T1).

C. Upper extremity muscle innervation. Because most muscles are innervated by multiple segments, it is necessary to know all the roots controlling a given muscle. Figure 1-4 indicates the roots contributing to a given muscle in the upper extremity. For purposes of strength grading, the following 5-point scale has been adopted by the American Academy of Orthopedic Surgeons.

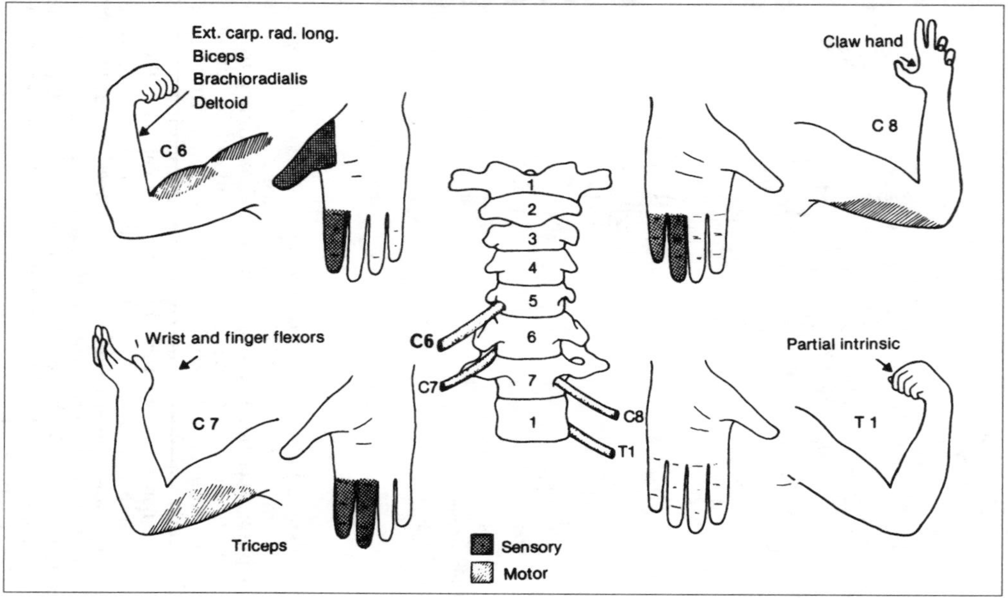

Fig. 1-3. Sensory and motor innervation C6–T1. Note: Only sensory loss is shown in the shaded hand and only muscle involvement is shown in the arm. (Reproduced with permission from DJ McQueen. The Cervical Spine. In HH Sherk [ed], *Neurologic Evaluation* [2nd ed]. Philadelphia: Lippincott, 1989. P 206.)

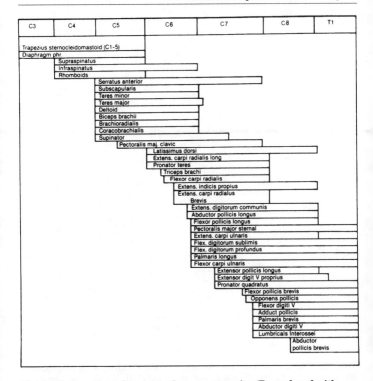

Fig. 1-4. Innervation of muscles of upper extremity. (Reproduced with permission from L Guttman. *Spinal Cord Injuries: Comprehensive Management and Research.* Oxford, England: Blackwell, 1973. Pp ix, 694.)

Grade	Level of strength
1	Flicker
2	Less than antigravity
3	Maintains position against gravity
4	Moves against submaximal resistance
5	Full strength

D. Brachial plexus structure. Unless a physician works with the brachial plexus constantly, it is difficult to remember its anatomy accurately. The anatomy is depicted in Figure 1-5 to aid in understanding injuries from birth and later trauma. Most traction injuries involve the upper roots.

E. Lower extremity motor innervation. Knowledge of lower extremity motor innervation is important for understanding spina bifida, lumbar disc herniation, spinal cord injury, and other conditions. Innervation of muscles generally corresponds to descending spinal segments, with the notable exceptions of the gluteus maximus, medius, and minimus (L5–S2).

The most important motors to know are iliopsoas (L1–L3), adductors (L2-4), quadriceps (L2–L4), hamstrings

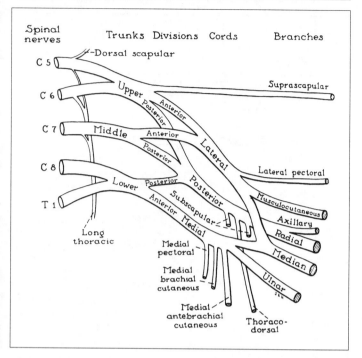

Fig. 1-5. Structure of the brachial plexus. (Reproduced with permission from WH Hollinshead. *Anatomy for Surgeons* [3rd ed]. Philadelphia: Lippincott, 1982. P 221.)

(L4–L5), anterior tibialis (L4–L5), gastrocnemius (S1), and glutei (L5–S2), shown in Figure 1-6.

III. Skeletal development

A. Appearance of secondary ossification centers and physeal closure. In many situations it is important to know whether an epiphysis should be ossified at a given age, such as in evaluating a patient with a hip dislocation, skeletal dysplasia, or elbow fracture. Normal times for appearance of secondary ossification and physeal closure of the long bones are given in Figure 1-7 and for the hand and foot in Figure 1-8.

Some observations deserve special mention:

1. The distal femoral epiphysis is the first to ossify, at approximately 39 weeks' gestation; the proximal tibia ossifies 1 week later.

2. The mean time for ossification of the proximal femoral epiphysis is 4 months, but any point up to 11 months may be normal. The greater trochanter ossifies at 4–6 years.

3. The triradiate cartilage closes before the iliac crest reaches Risser I (begins ossifying).

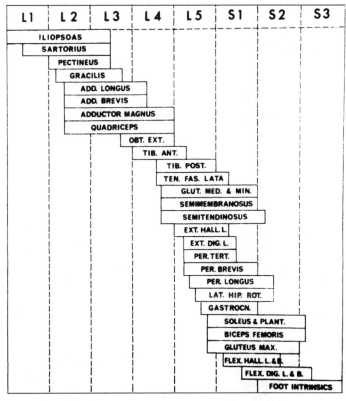

L1	L2	L3	L4	L5	S1	S2	S3

ILIOPSOAS
SARTORIUS
PECTINEUS
GRACILIS
ADD. LONGUS
ADD. BREVIS
ADDUCTOR MAGNUS
QUADRICEPS
OBT. EXT.
TIB. ANT.
TIB. POST.
TEN. FAS. LATA
GLUT. MED. & MIN.
SEMIMEMBRANOSUS
SEMITENDINOSUS
EXT. HALL. L.
EXT. DIG. L.
PER. TERT.
PER. BREVIS
PER. LONGUS
LAT. HIP. ROT.
GASTROCN.
SOLEUS & PLANT.
BICEPS FEMORIS
GLUTEUS MAX.
FLEX. HALL. L. & B.
FLEX. DIG. L. & B.
FOOT INTRINSICS

Fig. 1-6. Segmental innervation of muscles of the lower limb.
(Reproduced with permission from WJW Sharrard. Orthopaedic
surgery of spina bifida. *Clin Orthop* 92:196, 1972.)

4. The tarsal navicular does not ossify until 3–4 years, so
   its location must be inferred from the position of the
   first metatarsal.
5. The last physis to close is that of the medial clavicle, at
   20–25 years.
6. The sequence of ossification about the elbow can be
   remembered by the mnemonic **CRITOE** (Fig. 1-9):

   Capitellum (age 2)
   Radial head (age 5)
   Internal epicondyle (age 7)
   Trochlea (age 9)
   Olecranon (age 10)
   External epicondyle (age 11)

7. **Angle of distal humeral articular surface.** This
   angle is key to understanding any angular change about

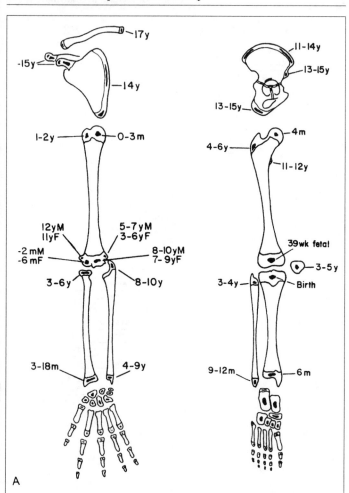

Fig. 1-7. Age of appearance (A) of secondary ossification centers and physeal closure (B) in the long bones. (Reproduced with permission from JA Ogden. *Skeletal Injury in the Child* [2nd ed]. Philadelphia: Saunders, 1990. P 84.)

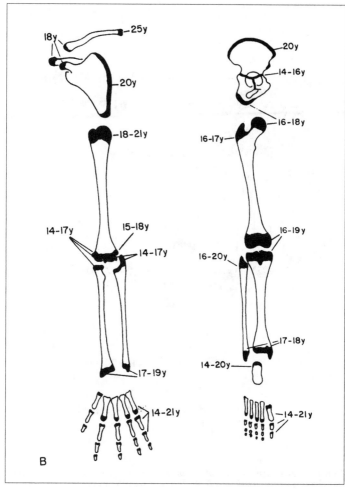

Fig. 1-7. *(continued)*

the elbow. It is best measured by the Baumann angle, between the humeral shaft and the lateral condylar physis (Fig. 1-10). Its normal value is 72 degrees ± 4 degrees. There is no difference between sexes or ages from 2 to 13 years.

B. Cervical spine radiographic normal values for children (Fig. 1-11)

1. The cervical spine in children is characterized by increased mobility at C2–C3, termed **pseudosubluxation**. This mobility should not exceed 3 mm.
2. The tip of the odontoid should be no more than 1 cm from the basion of the skull.

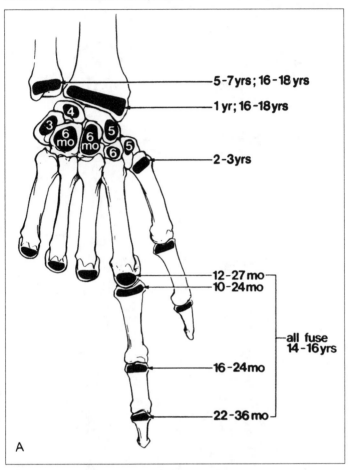

Fig. 1-8. Age of appearance of secondary ossification centers and physeal closure in the hand and foot. (m.i.u. = months in utero.) (Part A reproduced with permission from CA Rockwood Jr, D Green. *Fractures in Children* [3rd ed]. Philadelphia: Lippincott, 1991. P 320; Part B from JT Aitken, J Joseph. *A Manual of Human Anatomy* [2nd ed]. Edinburgh: Livingstone, 1966. P 80.)

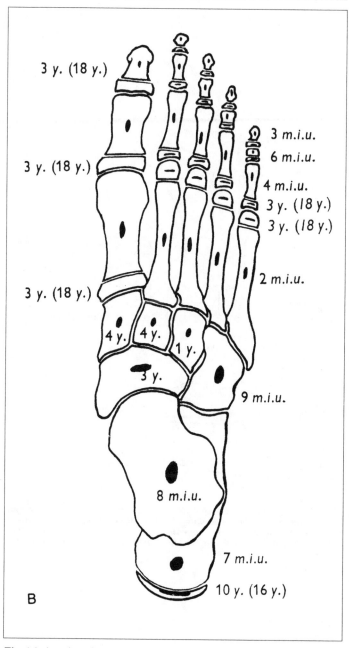

Fig. 1-8. *(continued)*

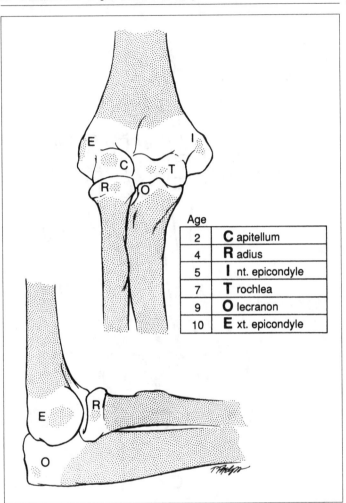

Age		
2	**C**	apitellum
4	**R**	adius
5	**I**	nt. epicondyle
7	**T**	rochlea
9	**O**	lecranon
10	**E**	xt. epicondyle

Fig. 1-9. Age of appearance of ossification centers about the elbow can be summarized by the mnemonic CRITOE. (Reproduced with permission from PD Sponseller. Orthopedic Injuries. In DG Nichols [ed], *The Handbook of Advanced Pediatric Life Support.* St. Louis: Mosby, 1991. P 350.)

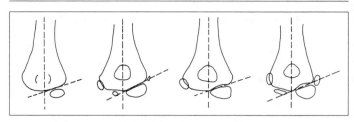

Fig. 1-10. Variations in the configuration of the distal humerus and landmarks used for measurement of the Baumann angle. (Reproduced with permission from DM Williamson et al. Normal characteristics of the Baumann angle. *J Pediatr Orthop* 12:636, 1992.)

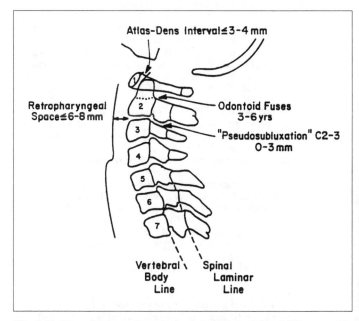

Fig. 1-11. Normal values of cervical spine alignment for children age 10 and younger. (Reproduced with permission from PD Sponseller. Orthopedic Injuries. In DG Nichols [ed], *The Handbook of Advanced Pediatric Life Support*. St. Louis: Mosby 1991. P 353.)

3. The physis of the odontoid normally fuses between 3 and 6 years.
4. The atlas-dens interval should be less than or equal to 3–4 mm or less.
5. The Powers ratio is the ratio of the distance from basion to posterior arch of C1 divided by the distance from the opisthion to the anterior arch of C1. It should be less than 1.
6. The retropharyngeal space should not exceed 8 mm; if greater, it could signify bleeding from a fracture or a dislocation.
7. The spinal laminae should form a smooth line posteriorly.
8. The vertebral bodies may be wedged anteriorly, especially on their superior surfaces, until age 10.

C. **Development of the cervical spine** (Fig. 1-12)
   1. **First cervical vertebra (atlas)**
      a. The vertebral **body** (A) is not ossified at birth. The center (occasionally two centers) appears during the first year after birth. The body may fail to develop, and forward extension of the neural arches may take its place.
      b. **Neural arches** (C) appear bilaterally at approximately the seventh fetal week. Most of the anterior portion of the superior articulating surface is usually formed by the body.
      c. The **synchondrosis of spinous processes** (D) unites by the third year. Union may rarely be preceded by the appearance of a secondary center within the synchondrosis.
      d. The **neurocentral synchondrosis** (F) fuses at approximately the seventh year.
      e. The **ligament surrounding the superior vertebral notch** (K) may ossify, especially later in life.
   2. **Second cervical vertebra (axis)** (Fig. 1-13)
      a. In the **body** (A) of the axis, one center (occasionally two) appears by the fifth fetal month.
      b. **Neural arches** (C) appear bilaterally by the seventh fetal month.
      c. **Neural arches** (D) fuse posteriorly by the second or third year.
      d. Occasionally, a secondary center is present in each **bifid tip of the spinous process** (E).
      e. The **neurocentral synchondrosis** (F) fuses at 3–6 years.
      f. The **inferior epiphyseal ring** (G) appears at puberty and fuses at approximately 25 years.
      g. The **"summit" ossification center** (H) for the odontoid appears at 3–6 years and fuses with the odontoid by 12 years.
      h. In the **odontoid (dens)** (I), two centers appear by the fifth fetal month and fuse with each other by the seventh month.
      i. The **synchondrosis between the odontoid and the neural arch** (J) fuses at 3–6 years.
      j. The **synchondrosis between the odontoid and the body** (L) fuses at 3–6 years.
      k. The **posterior surface of body and odontoid** (M).

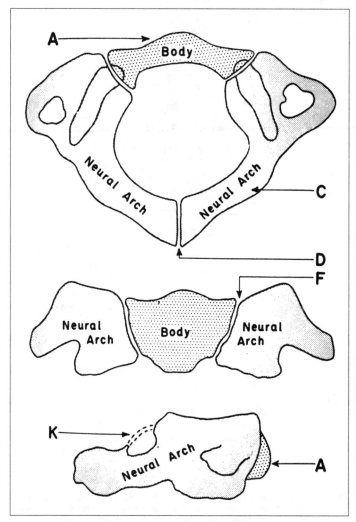

Fig. 1-12. Normal development of C1 (atlas) in children. (A = body; C = neural arches; D = synchondrosis of spinous processes; F = neuro-central synchondrosis; K = ligament around the superior vertebral notch.) (Reproduced with permission from DK Bailey. Normal cervical spine in infants and children. *Radiology* 59:713, 1952.)

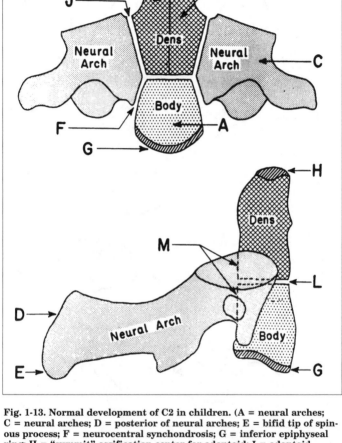

Fig. 1-13. Normal development of C2 in children. (A = neural arches; C = neural arches; D = posterior of neural arches; E = bifid tip of spinous process; F = neurocentral synchondrosis; G = inferior epiphyseal ring; H = "summit" ossification center for odontoid; I = odontoid (dens); J = synchondrosis between odontoid and neural arch; L = synchondrosis between odontoid and body; M = posterior surfaces of odontoid and body.) (Reproduced with permission from DK Bailey. Normal cervical spine in infants and children. *Radiology* 59:713, 1952.)

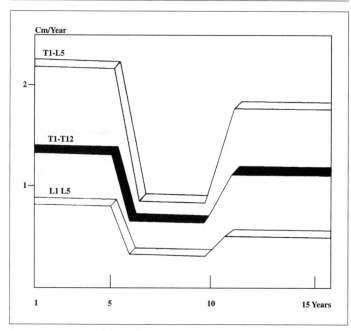

Fig. 1-14. Approximate growth velocity of the spine by segments: thoracic, lumbar and combined segments. Note that the greatest velocity is in preschool years, after which a significant drop occurs. (Reproduced with permission from A Dimeglio. Growth of the spine before five years. *J Pediatr Orthop* 1:102, 1993.)

D. Spinal growth (Fig. 1-14)
  1. The growth of the spine takes place earlier than that of the extremities, but not as early as cranial growth.
  2. **Guidelines.** These guidelines are useful in predicting the consequences for growth after arthrodesis or a related procedure is performed in a growing child.
     a. T1–S1 growth rates:

        | 0–5 yrs: | 2 cm/yr |
        | 6–10 yrs: | 0.9 cm/yr |
        | 10 yrs: | 1.8 cm/yr through growth spurt |

     b. Growth of the T1–S1 segment is two-thirds complete by age 5.
     c. Growth remaining from T1–S1 at age 5 is 15 cm.
     d. **Note: Posterior arthrodesis alone does not stop growth completely within a fused segment.** Further growth can cause relative compression of disc space, exacerbation of preexisting lordosis, or "crankshaft" rotation of scoliosis.

3. Growth remaining calculation

0.07 cm × number of spinal segments × growth years left

For example, thoracolumbar spinal growth in a girl at age 10 = 0.07 × 17 segments × 4 years = 1.2 × 4 = 4.8 cm.

4. Figure 1-15 displays graphs to use in calculating remaining growth by spinal segment for boys (A) and for girls (B).

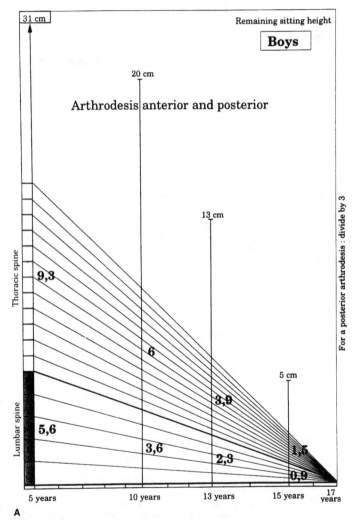

A

Fig. 1-15. Growth remaining in the spine by segment (A) for boys, (B) for girls. Note that the remaining component of sitting height is composed of head, cervical spine, and cranium. (Reproduced with permission from A Dimeglio. Growth of the spine before five years. *J Pediatr Orthop* 1:102, 1993.)

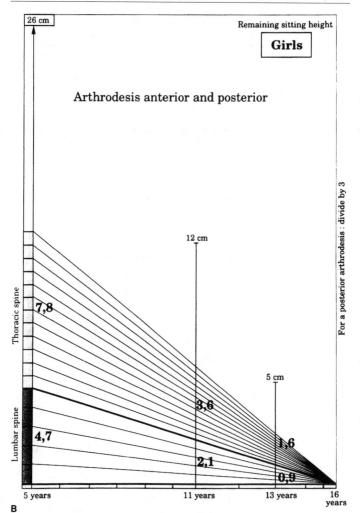

B

Fig. 1-15. *(continued)*

E. Extremity growth. Relative contributions to the growth of the long bones are shown in Figure 1-16.

1. The contribution of each physis to longitudinal growth is a reflection of its activity, which in turn influences remodeling potential. A simple rule of thumb is that **most growth occurs away from the elbow and at the knee** in the upper and lower extremities, respectively.

2. **Estimating growth**

   a. At each physis, growth during the preadolescent years can be estimated using these approximate figures:

Proximal femur	⅛ in./yr
Distal femur	⅜ in./yr
Proximal tibia	¼ in./yr
Distal tibia	³⁄₁₆ in./yr

   These estimates hold true until age 13 for girls and age 15 for boys. For long growth periods of more than 3 years, it is better to consult growth tables (Figure 1-17).

   b. Total adult height = 2 × height at age 2.

   c. Total adult length of lower extremities = 2 × length at age 4.

   d. Growth ceases in girls at 15–15½ years, in boys at 17–18 years.

   e. Another way to estimate adult height:

$$\text{Males} = \frac{\text{father's height} + \text{mother's height} + 6 \text{ cm}}{2}$$

$$\text{Females} = \frac{\text{father's height} + \text{mother's height} - 6 \text{ cm}}{2}$$

Two standard deviations = ±5 cm

3. **Growth curves for long bones.** These are useful when absolute lengths are needed. Figures 1-18 and 1-19 show normal growth curves in boys and girls.

4. **Growth remaining curves** (Fig. 1-20). These are a reformulation of the data shown in Figures 1-18 and 1-19. The format shown in Figure 1-20 is especially useful for estimating the effects of physeal closure. The physician must know the patient's skeletal age and percentile rank for height (see Figs. 1-18 and 1-19). The percentile rank is indicated by plotting points for a given skeletal age with respect to the mean the ± 1 and ± 2 S.D. lines.

5. **Longitudinal growth from distal tibial physes** (see Fig. 1-20).

   a. Distal tibial and fibular physeal fractures often occur in childhood and adolescence. Growth plate damage may occur as a result of these fractures. Physeal closure in either bone must then be evaluated for its significance in future shortening and angular deformity.

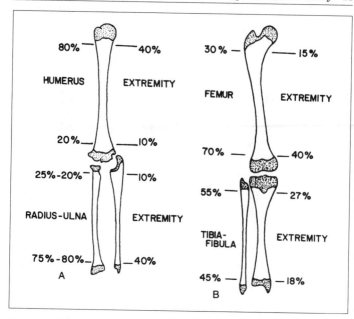

Fig. 1-16. Relative contributions to growth of the long bones of the arm (A) and the leg (B). (Reproduced with permission from JA Ogden. *Skeletal Injury in the Child* [2nd ed]. Philadelphia: Saunders, 1990. P 85.)

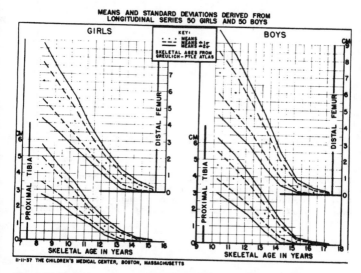

Fig. 1-17. Growth remaining in normal distal femur and proximal tibia following consecutive skeletal age levels. (Reproduced with permission from M Anderson. Growth and predictions of growth in the lower extremities. *J Bone Joint Surg [Am]* 45:1, 1963.)

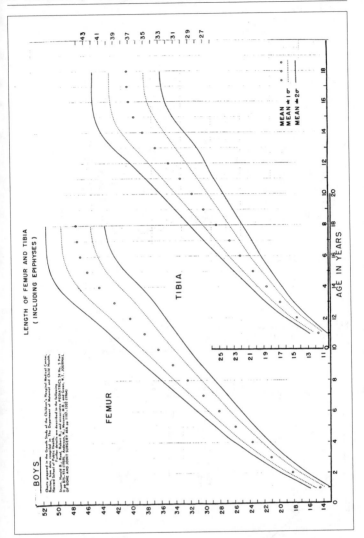

Fig. 1-18. Length of normal femur and tibia for boys (including epiphyses). (Reproduced with permission from M Anderson, MB Messner, WT Green. Distribution of lengths of the normal femur and tibia in children from one to eighteen years of age. *J Bone Joint Surg [Am]* 46:1197, 1964.)

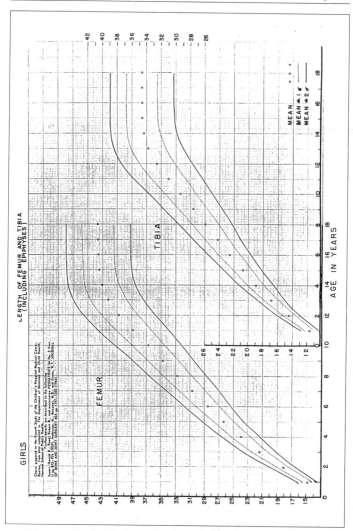

Fig. 1-19. Length of normal femur and tibia for girls (including epiphyses). (Reproduced with permission from M Anderson, MB Messner, WT Green. Distribution of lengths of the normal femur and tibia in children from one to eighteen years of age. *J Bone Joint Surg [Am]* 46:1197, 1964.)

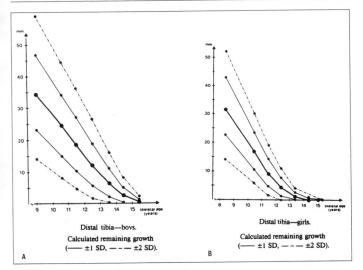

Fig. 1-20. Growth remaining in distal tibia (mean ± 2 SD) for boys (A) and girls (B). (Reproduced with permission from J Karrholm. Growth of distal tibial physis. *Clin Orthop* 191:121, 1984.)

      b. The growth-remaining graphs in Figure 1-20 may be used to predict the deformity. The line to follow for a given patient may be obtained from the existing length of the tibia with respect to the mean and ± 1–2 S.D. as seen in Figures 1-18 and 1-19.

      c. Length lost from total growth arrest may be calculated. In general, inequality of less than 1 cm is of no clinical significance.

      d. Prediction of angular growth disturbance as a result of peripheral arrest may be calculated from the growth remaining and the width of the physis. Because the average distal tibia is 4–5 cm in width, 10 degrees of angulation is unlikely to occur in boys after the age of 13½; in girls after age 11½. This also applies to hemiepiphyseodesis.

6. Straight-line graph for predictions of discrepancy. For growth disturbances that do not change characteristics over time, the eventual limb length inequality at maturity may be calculated by plotting data points on the straight-line graph developed by Mosely (Fig. 1-21), if the skeletal age is known. The procedure is explained step by step in Figure 1-22. Conditions for which the graph may not be appropriate are those with a phasic nature, such as discrepancy due to juvenile rheumatoid arthritis or Klippel-Trenaunay syndrome.

7. Upper-extremity growth. Growth arrest occurs less commonly in the upper extremity. Occasionally, however, due to infection, tumor, or trauma, growth may be

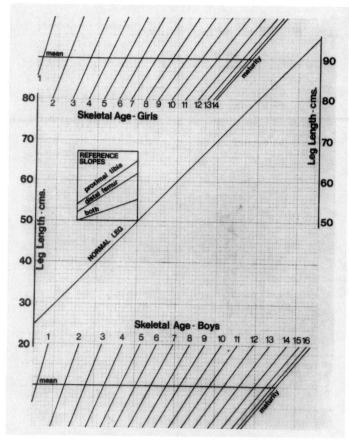

Fig. 1-21. Moseley straight-line graph for predicting limb length inequality. (Reproduced with permission from CF Moseley. A straight line graph for prediction of leg length discrepancies. *J Bone Joint Surg [Am]* 59A:176, 1977.)

affected, and it may become necessary to calculate the resulting discrepancy in limb length. In such cases, growth remaining curves for the upper extremities (Fig. 1-23) are useful.

8. **Overall physical growth norms** include mean stature and weight for age and their percentiles, for both sexes (Fig. 1-24). These overall growth norms are useful in screening for growth disturbances and estimating height at maturity.

F. **Alignment in the transverse plane**
   1. **Femoral anteversion**
      a. Femoral anteversion is the angle between the plane

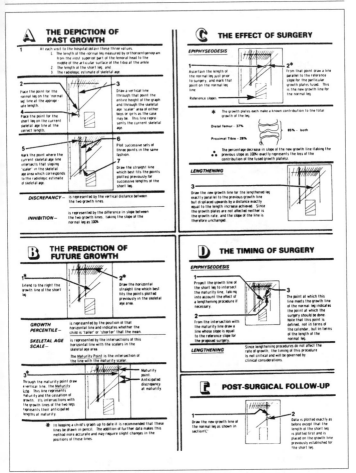

Fig. 1-22. Instructions for the Moseley graph. (Reproduced with permission from CF Moseley. A straight-line graph for prediction for leg-length discrepancies. *J Bone Joint Surg [Am]* 59:174, 1977.)

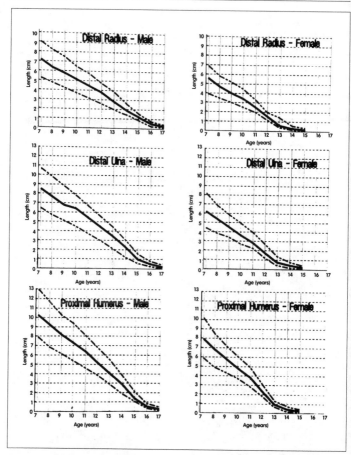

Fig. 1-23. Growth remaining from major upper extremity physes: These are graphs from the Child Research Council, Denver, Colo. Mean *(solid line)* and two standard deviations *(dotted lines)*. (Reproduced from DT Bortel, JW Pritchett. Straight line graphs for the prediction of growth of the upper extremities. *J Bone Joint Surg [Am]* 75:885, 1993.)

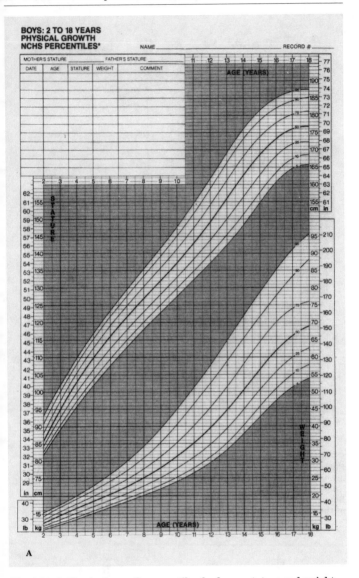

Fig. 1-24. A. Physical growth percentiles for boys—stature and weight. B. Physical growth percentiles for girls—stature and weight. (Reproduced with permission from PVV Hamill. Prediction of growth. *Am J Clin Nutr* 32:607, 1979.)

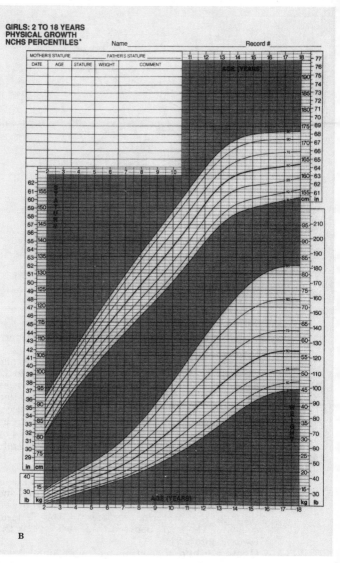

Fig. 1-24. *(continued)*

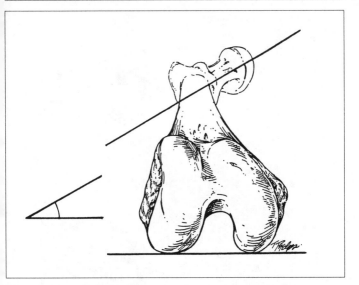

Fig. 1-25. Femoral anteversion.

of the femoral head and neck and that of the posterior surface of the femoral condyles (Fig. 1-25).

Femoral anteversion declines steadily in normal children from a mean of 25 degrees at birth to 15 degrees at adulthood (Fig. 1-26). It may be followed clinically by recording internal and external rotation of the hip in extension. Anteversion is most accurately measured by CT scan. The method of Murphy is shown here. Anteversion may also be measured by standard radiographs using the techniques of Ogate or Magilligan.

b. The **Murphy method** (CT measurement of anteversion). On sequential cuts made by CT scan, a line is drawn through the centers of the femoral head and base of the neck (Fig. 1-27). Another line is drawn through the posterior surfaces of the femoral condyles. The angle between these two lines is the femoral anteversion.

c. **Ogate method** of determining femoral anteversion using biplane radiographs.

  (1) The Ogate method may be used **when CT is not readily available.** It uses graphs to provide trigonometric calculations of anteversion as well as true neck-shaft angle from two standardized plain radiographs. The Ogate method is based on the fact that the tibia is perpendicular to the condylar axis when the knee is flexed. The method is accurate when positioning is done carefully, to within ± 6 degrees for antev-

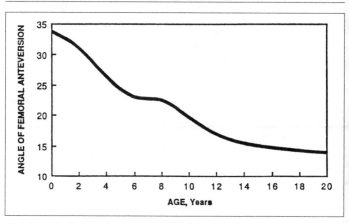

Fig. 1-26. Normal values for femoral anteversion from birth to adulthood. (Reproduced with permission from AR Shands, MK Steele. Torsion of the femur. *J Bone Joint Surg [Am]* 40:803, 1958.)

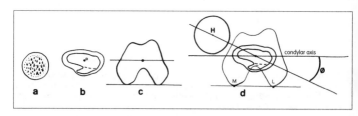

Fig. 1-27. Measurement of anteversion by CT scan. (a) Center of femoral head; (b) center of base of femoral neck; (c) line through posterior aspect of femoral condyles; (d) anteversion (θ) is the angle between the two lines so defined. If the femoral head is posterior to the condylar axis, the value of the angle is negative and is termed retroversion. (H = center femoral head; M = medial femoral condyle; L = lateral femoral condyle.) (Reproduced with permission from SB Murphy. Femoral anteversion. *J Bone Joint Surg [Am]* 69:1175, 1987.)

ersion and within ± 5 degrees for true neck-shaft angle.

(2) **Technique for obtaining radiographs.** The patient is positioned with the knee flexed 90 degrees and perpendicular to the surface of the x-ray table (Fig. 1-28). This places the condylar plane of the femur in a true horizontal position. A **projected anteroposterior neck-shaft x-ray** is taken, and the angle is drawn and labeled alpha.

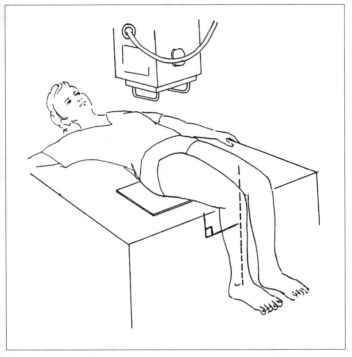

Fig. 1-28. Positioning for the projected anteroposterior neck-shaft x-ray in the Ogate method of determining femoral anteversion. The projected neck-shaft angle obtained on the radiograph (alpha) is used in the next step (see Figs. 1-30 and 1-31).

The patient is then positioned on the side, with the knee flexed and the tibia horizontal (Fig. 1-29). A **projected lateral neck-shaft** x-ray is taken, and the angle is drawn and labeled beta.

(3) Using the graphs in Figures 1-30 and 1-31, values for true neck-shaft angle and anteversion may be obtained.

G. Coronal plane alignment

1. The coronal tibiofemoral angle changes dramatically during the first 5 years of life: from varus to excessive valgus to "normal" valgus angle. Salenius' graph (redrawn in Fig. 1-32) best illustrates normal development. Data for the graph were taken from clinical measurements of 1,000 normal children. Radiographs are not generally necessary in the first 12–18 months of life. (Chap. 2 details the interpretation of abnormal conditions.)

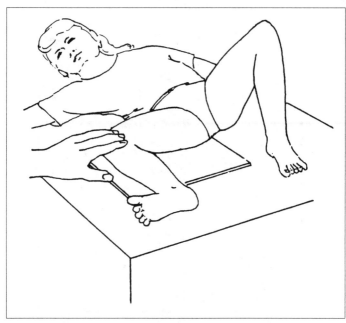

Fig. 1-29. Positioning for the projected lateral neck shaft x-ray in the Ogate method. The tibia should rest freely flat on the cassette. The projected neck-shaft angle obtained (beta) is used in the next step (see Figs. 1-30 and 1-31).

2. **Alignment of the lower extremity**
   a. Knowledge of normal tibiofemoral alignment is essential for planning osteotomies about the knee. Normal values vary slightly, depending on the width of the pelvis and the lengths of the limbs.
   b. The **mechanical axis** is the angle of the two lines between the centers of the hip and the knee and centers of the knee and the ankle. The normal angle is 0 degrees, inclined 3 degrees from the vertical (Fig. 1-33).
   c. The **anatomic axis** is the angle between the tibial and femoral diaphyses; normal is 6 degrees.
   d. The **knee joint line,** defined by the medial and lateral femoral condyles, should be horizontal.
   e. The **femoral joint angle,** or the angle between the anatomic femoral axis and the joint line, is $90 - (\beta + \theta)$.
   f. The **tibial joint angle,** or the angle between the anatomic tibial axis and the joint line, is $90 - \theta$.
H. **Clinical evaluation of rotation of the lower extremities.** Rotational abnormalities of the lower extremities can be approached in a systematic fashion. The **foot progression angle** quantifies the sum of rota-

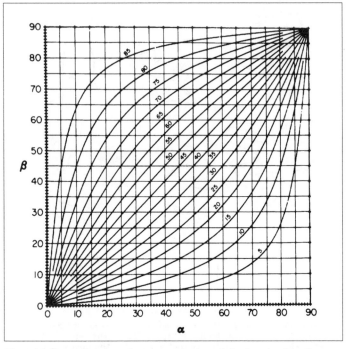

Fig. 1-30. Determination of true anteversion of the femur using the intersection of projected anteroposterior (alpha) and lateral (beta) angles (see Figs. 1-28 and 1-29). (Reproduced with permission from K Ogate. A simple biplane method of measuring femoral anteversion and neck-shaft angle. *J Bone Joint Surg [Am]* 61:846, 1979.)

tions occurring in the femur, tibia, and foot. These components may be assessed by the parameters defined here. Normal values throughout growth, as determined by Staheli and colleagues, are given for all these parameters. Treatment for rotational deformities is rarely indicated, but showing the natural progression to the parents in graphic form can be helpful.

1. **Metatarsal adduction** (Fig. 1-34). Forefoot adduction (deviation toward the body midline) is generally recorded from clinical measurements, but radiographic norms are available. Metatarsal adduction can be quantified by drawing a line through the heel bisector and noting which toe it intersects (Fig. 1-35). Normally, this line falls between the second and third toes. Moderate to severe adduction is present when the line falls lateral to the fourth toe.

2. **Foot progression angle.** The foot progression angle is the end product of all rotational components in the

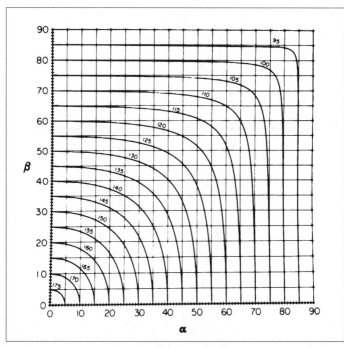

Fig. 1-31. Determination of true neck-shaft angle. (Reproduced with permission from K Ogate. A simple biplane method of measuring femoral anteversion and neck-shaft angle. *J Bone Joint Surg [Am]* 61:846, 1979.)

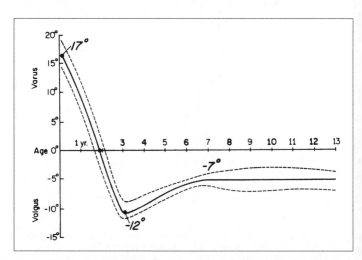

Fig. 1-32. The tibiofemoral angle during growth. (Reproduced with permission from P Salenius. The development of the tibiofemoral angle in children. *J Bone Joint Surg [Am]* 57:260, 1975.)

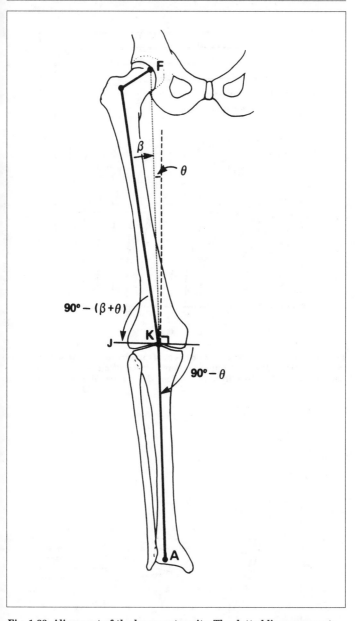

Fig. 1-33. Alignment of the lower extremity. The dotted line represents the mechanical axis; dashed line, the vertical axis; and solid lines, the anatomic axis. In normal subjects, beta = 6 degrees and theta = 3 degrees, but these may vary depending on distance between hip centers, femoral neck-shaft angle, and limb length. (A = center of ankle; F = center of hip; J = joint line; K = center of knee.)

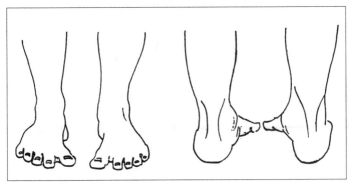

Fig. 1-34. Appearance of metatarsus adductus.

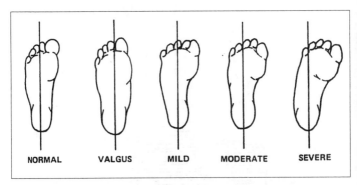

Fig. 1-35. Quantification of metatarsus adductus. This is done with the child prone. A line is drawn down the midline of the heel and the examiner notes which toe it intersects. (Reproduced with permission from EE Bleck. Developmental orthopaedics. III: Toddlers. *Dev Med Child Neuro* 24:533, 1982.)

lower extremity: hip, femur, knee, tibia, and foot. It is the angle formed by the position of the foot (on average) with the direction of walking (Fig. 1-36, *top*).

3. The **thigh-foot angle** is an approximate clinical measure of tibial torsion or foot malrotation. It is assessed with the patient prone and the ankle gently dorsiflexed to a neutral position (Fig. 1-36, *bottom*). Normal values with age are given in Figure 1-37A.

4. Unlike the thigh-foot angle, the **transmalleolar axis** reflects rotation within the tibia or fibula alone. The transmalleolar axis is assessed with the patient prone and a line drawn between the medial and lateral malleoli (Fig. 1-37B).

5. Internal (medial) and external (lateral) **rotation of the hip** in extension are used to assess the relative con-

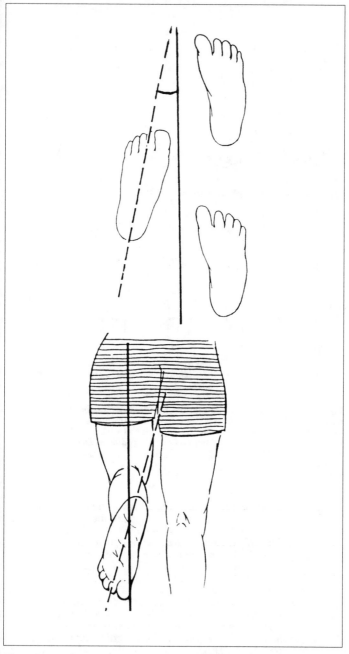

Fig. 1-36. The foot progression angle *(top)*, and the thigh-foot angle *(bottom)*.

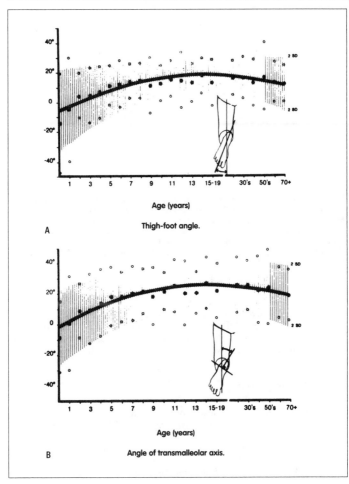

Fig. 1-37. A. Normal values for the thigh-foot angle with age. **B.** Normal values for the transmalleolar axis with age. (Reproduced with permission from LT Staheli. Lower extremity rotational problems in children. *J Bone Joint Surg [Am]* 67:39, 1985.)

tributions of the hip to rotation (Fig. 1-38A, B). Anteversion is likely to be present if internal rotation exceeds 70 degrees and external rotation is less than 20 degrees. Graphs of the normal range with age are given in Figure 1-38C and D.

I. **Normal radiographic measurements of the pediatric foot.** Radiographs are helpful in interpreting pathology in both the unoperated and the postoperative foot. The films should be taken with the patient standing, if possible. Normal values are given for the lateral talocalcaneal angle in

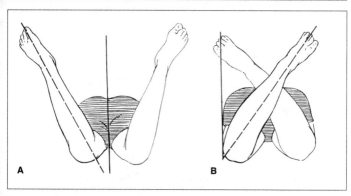

Fig. 1-38. Hip rotation is usually measured in extension for assessment of torsion deformities. A. Measurement of internal rotation. B. Measurement of external rotation. C. Normal values for internal rotation with age (female). D. Normal values for external rotation with age (both sexes). (Parts C and D reproduced with permission from LT Staheli. Lower extremity rotational problems in children. *J Bone Joint Surg [Am]* 67:39, 1985.)

Figure 1-39A and for the anteroposterior talocalcaneal angle in Figure 1-39B. Note that a decline in value of both angles is seen with a varus foot (increasing parallelism) and an increase is seen with a valgus foot (increasing divergence).

Bibliography

Magilligan DJ. Calculation of the angle of anteversion by means of horizontal lateral roentgenography. *J Bone Joint Surg [Am]* 38:1231, 1956.

Murphy SB. Femoral anteversion. *J Bone Joint Surg [Am]* 69:1169, 1987.

Tyshetz F. *Pediatric Endocrinology.* New York: Dekker, 1990.

IV. Normal gait in children. Virtually all aspects of normal gait can be thought of as being integrated to minimize energy consumption. Gait deviations occur in response to a patient's neurologic or mechanical abnormalities. To understand gait by visual or laboratory analysis, it must be broken down into component characteristics.

A. Definitions

 1. Kinematics: the study of motion.

 2. Kinetics: the study of the forces that produce movement.

 3. Cadence: number of steps per unit of time.

 4. Stride: one cycle, including right and left steps.

 5. Stance phase: the period when one or both feet are on the ground.

 6. First rocker: the first stage of ankle motion in stance, from heel strike to foot flat; decelerates inertia of body;

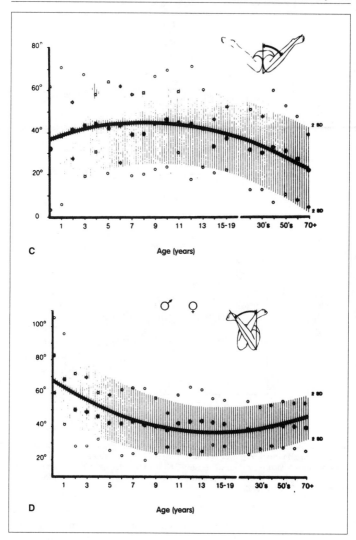

Fig. 1-38. *(continued)*

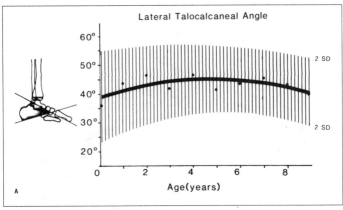

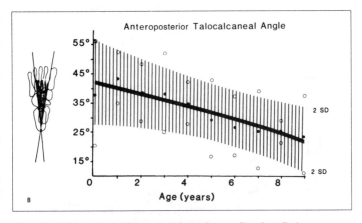

Fig. 1-39. A. Lateral talocalcaneal angle in the standing foot. B. Anteroposterior talocalcaneal angle in the standing foot. (Reproduced with permission from RA Vanderwilde, LT Staheli, Chew DE, Malagon V. Measurements on radiographs of the foot in normal infants and children. *J Bone Joint Surg [Am]* 70:407, 1988.)

tibialis anterior contracts eccentrically, elongating slowly to prevent foot slap.

7. **Second rocker**: from foot flat to heel rise; deceleration of tibia to relax quadriceps; soleus contracts eccentrically, elongating slowly to prevent knee buckling.

8. **Third rocker**: from heel rise to toe off the ground; accelerates limb; gastrocnemius and soleus contract concentrically, shortening to provide push-off.

9. Normal walking gait is 60% **stance** and 40% **swing**; therefore, 20% of time during walking is spent in **double support** (both feet on the ground). Figures 1-40 and 1-41 show the phases of the gait cycle.

B. **Normal parameters**

1. **Mature gait** is fully developed by age 7.

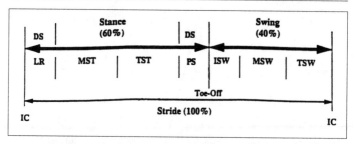

Fig. 1-40. Phases of gait cycle. (DS = double support, LR = loading response, MST = midstance, TST = terminal stance, PS = preswing, ISW = initial swing, MSW = midswing, TSW = terminal swing, IC = initial contact.

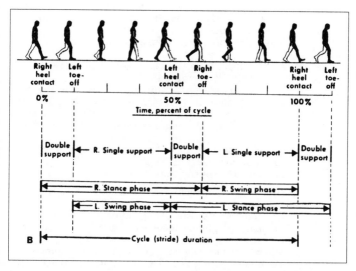

Fig. 1-41. Phases of gait cycle illustrated with figures. (Reproduced with permission from V Inman. *Human Walking*. Baltimore: Williams & Wilkins, 1981.)

2. Velocity

2 yrs:	0.78 m/sec ± 0.2
4 yrs:	1.0 m/sec ± 0.2
6 yrs:	1.1 m/sec ± 0.2
Adult:	1.5 m/sec ± 0.2

3. Cadence

2 yrs:	180 steps/min
4 yrs:	160 steps/min
Adult:	116 steps/min

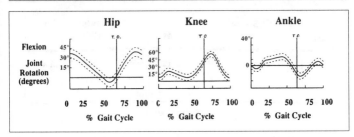

Fig. 1-42. Normal joint kinematics at the hip, knee, and ankle. (t.o. = toe-off.) (Reproduced with permission from JR Gage. Clinical use of kinetics for evaluation of pathological gait in cerebral palsy. *J Bone Joint Surg [Am]* **76:626, 1994.)**

4. **Hip flexion and extension** ranges from 0 to 40 degrees during normal walking. Figure 1-42 shows separate graphs of normal joint motion during gait for hip, knee, and ankle.
5. **Knee flexion and extension** ranges from 5 to 60 degrees.
6. **Ankle** ranges from –5 to 20 degrees plantar flexion.

C. **Muscle activity during gait**

1. Normal muscle activity while walking may be measured by surface electrodes for large muscles and by fine wire electrodes for small muscles. Figure 1-43 provides a diagram showing which muscles are engaged at each phase of gait. Note that electromyographic data measure **muscle activity** (on/off) and **intensity** but not the **force of contraction**.
2. **Muscle control by phase**

Heel strike: gluteus maximus, hamstrings, tibialis anterior.

Loading response: hamstrings, tibialis anterior, quadriceps, gluteus medius and maximus, adductor magnus.

Midstance: soleus, quadriceps, gluteus maximus.

Terminal stance: soleus, gastrocnemius, peroneals, toe flexors.

Preswing: gastrocnemius, adductor longus, rectus femoris.

Initial swing: hip flexors, tibialis anterior, toe extensors.

Midswing: tibialis anterior.

Terminal swing: hamstrings, quadriceps, tibialis anterior.

Bibliography

Gage JR. *Gait Analysis in Cerebral Palsy*. London: MacKeith Press, 1991.

Gage JR. Clinical use of kinetics for evaluation of pathological gait in cerebral palsy. *J Bone Joint Surg [Am]* 76:622, 1994.

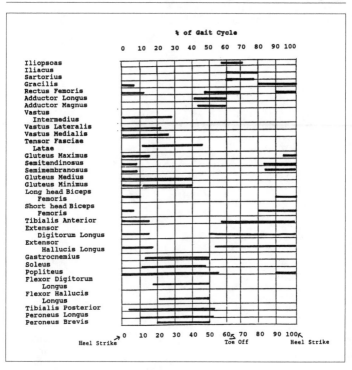

Fig. 1-43. Muscle activity during gait.

Abnormal Growth and Development

Selected pediatric orthopedic conditions are summarized here, with emphasis on central concepts and parameters. The goal is to provide working knowledge for treatment rather than specific treatment details, which are more extensively covered in standard texts. Also excluded here are genetic syndromes, neuromuscular disorders, and abnormal growth resulting from trauma, which are covered in other chapters.

Chapter Outline

I. Developmental dysplasia of the hip

A. Principles. Developmental dysplasia of the hip (DDH) is caused by forces acting on the hip in utero, and the risk is increased by abnormalities of connective tissue or the neurologic system. DDH represents a spectrum of disorders rather than a single condition, from hips which are subluxatable to dislocatable to dislocated. The combined incidence of these groups is 2–6 per 1,000 newborns.

All hips should be screened by a knowledgeable examiner at birth and again within the first few months of life.

B. Risk factors in history. The following factors increase the risk of hip dysplasia. Any of these factors should prompt re-examination or ultrasound.

1. Positive family history (10% are unstable).
2. Breech position at end of gestation (5% are unstable).
3. Large birth weight.

C. Physical examination for DDH in the newborn. The infant should be made as quiet and comfortable as possible for the examination, using warmth, physical contact, low light, feeding, or a pacifier. Abnormal physical signs, marked with an asterisk (*), should prompt ultrasound, with treatment if these are abnormal.

1. **Appearance at rest.** Affected side is more adducted at rest in unilateral cases and may have a deeper or extra high fold proximally.

*2. **Asymmetric passive abduction.** Dislocated hip cannot be passively abducted as far as the normal side (Fig. 2-1A).

*3. The **Barlow test** (posteriorly directed pressure on the adducted thigh) causes pistoning of the proximal femur if it is dislocatable (Fig. 2-1B).

*4. The **Ortolani test** (traction with abduction) causes a "clunk" as a dislocated hip is relocated. Examine each hip separately, stabilizing the pelvis with the other hand (Fig. 2-1C). Note that the Ortolani and Barlow tests are to detect **translation** of the femur. By itself, a click is not a positive test: Only 1% of patients with a click have dysplasia. A click may come from the patella or the meniscus of the knee as well as from the fascia lata or a synovial fold in the hip.

5. Proximal location of greater trochanters is a useful sign in diagnosing a patient with bilateral irreducible hip dislocations.

6. Significant foot deformity or torticollis may increase the risk of hip dysplasia and should prompt a careful examination of the hips.

D. Evaluation of the older child for DDH. In the older child with hip dysplasia, the signs change progressively. Reducibility is lost after about 3 months, and the physician must rely more on indirect signs to diagnose dysplasia:

1. Asymmetric range of passive abduction.
2. The **Galeazzi test** (adducting the flexed thighs together) shows thigh shortening on the side that is dislocated (Fig. 2-2A). The pelvis should be kept level during this test.
3. Leg length discrepancy.

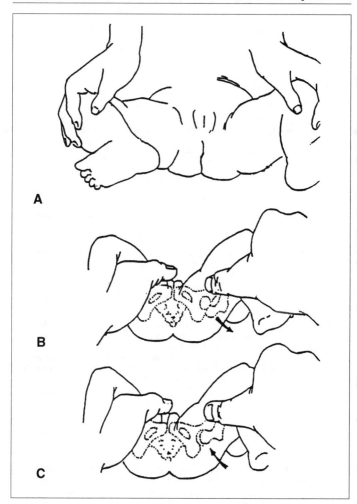

Fig. 2-1. Developmental hip dysplasia in the newborn. A. Asymmetric abduction, left side is dysplastic. B. Barlow test (done on one hip at a time). C. Ortolani test.

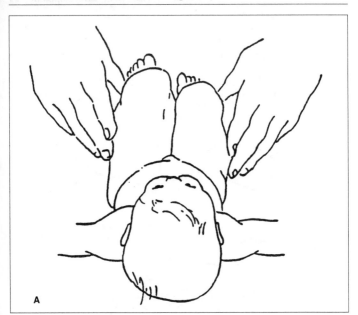

Fig. 2-2. Physical examination of newborn. A. The Galeazzi sign shows apparent thigh shortening on dysplastic side *(right)*. B. If dislocated, the greater trochanter lies proximal to Nélaton's line (anterior superior spine of the ilium to ischium). C. The Klisic line (between the greater trochanter and the anterior superior spine of the ilium) in the normal hip lies above the umbilicus.

    4. Trendelenburg gait (trunk lists toward the affected side each time weight is borne on it).
    5. Palpable femoral head posterior to the acetabulum.
    6. Nélaton's line (an imaginary line between the ischium and the anterior superior spine of the ilium) lies superior to the trochanter (Fig. 2-2B).
    7. Klisic's line—between the greater trochanter and the anterior superior spine of the ilium—projects cephalad to the umbilicus (Fig. 2-2C).
    8. Increased lumbar lordosis is present (if dysplasia is bilateral) due to posterior displacement and mechanical disadvantage of hip abductors.
  E. Ultrasound for hip dysplasia
    1. Principles. The precise role of ultrasound in diagnosis of dysplasia is still subject to significant regional variation. The main benefits of ultrasound are its ability to show cartilage and other soft tissue boundaries and to demonstrate stability in response to stress. In interpreting ultrasound results, consider both static and dynamic findings.

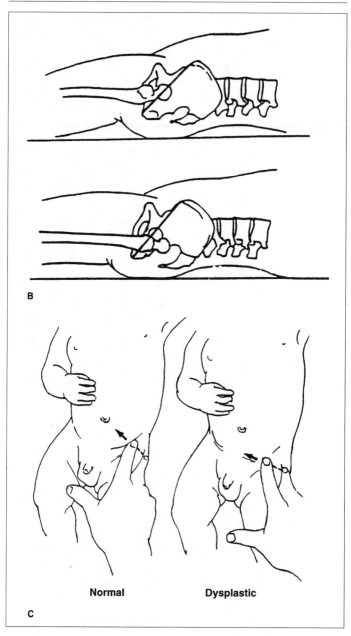

Normal   **Dysplastic**

C

Fig. 2-2. *(continued)*

The ultrasound view is named according to the direction of the transducer—transverse or coronal—and the position of the hip—neutral or flexed.

The highest frequency possible (3–7 MHz) gives the best resolution, but usually frequency must be reduced with increasing age to obtain adequate penetration.

2. **Coronal view.** In the coronal view, the landmarks are similar to those seen on a plain radiograph, when the transducer is in the midacetabular plane.

   a. The stability and gross appearance are the most important features.

   b. Other parameters to check are as follows (Fig. 2-3A):

   (1) Femoral head coverage, or percent of the femoral head medial to the outer line of the ilium. Normal femoral head coverage should be greater than 50% for boys, 44% for girls.

   (2) Alpha angle, or acetabular roof line, between the lateral ilium and the bony acetabular roof. It normally should be greater than 60 degrees.

   (3) Beta angle, or slope of the labrum versus the lateral wall of the ilium. It normally should be less than 55 degrees.

3. **Transverse view.** In the transverse view, the hip is flexed and the transducer is placed posterolaterally in the transverse plane of the body (Fig. 2-3B). The combination of echoes from the femoral metaphysis and the acetabulum normally form a U. When the hip is dislocated, the femoral head comes to lie lateral and posterior or to the acetabulum and the U is disrupted.

F. **Radiographic evaluation of hip dysplasia**

   1. The **grades of hip dislocation according to Tonnis** indicate the position of the ossific nucleus relative to Perkins' vertical line and Hilgenreiner's horizontal line (Fig. 2-4): (1) nucleus medial to Perkins' line, (2) nucleus lateral to Perkins' line, (3) nucleus at Hilgenreiner's line, (4) nucleus above Hilgenreiner's line.

   2. The **acetabular index** is the angle formed between Hilgenreiner's line and the inner and outer borders of the acetabular roof (Fig. 2-5A). It is useful in quantifying hip development in early years, before the center of the femoral head can be accurately identified. The normal values are shown in Figure 2-5B.

   3. **Center edge angle of Wiberg**

      a. The center edge angle (CEA) of Wiberg measures the coverage of the femoral head by the acetabulum (Fig. 2-6). Long-term follow-up studies by Wiberg have shown a correlation between development of symptoms after maturity and subnormal values of the CEA.

      b. CEA values for ages 5 through 13 (measurement is less precise under age 5):

Age	Lower limit of normal
5–8 yrs	19 degrees
9–12	25 degrees
13+	26 degrees

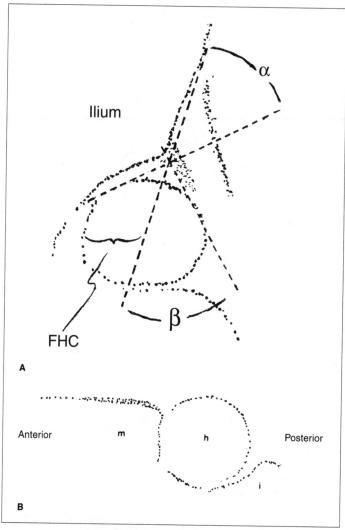

Fig. 2-3. Ultrasound for hip dysplasia. A. Coronal view in extension.
(FHC = femoral head coverage; alpha = acetabular roof line; beta =
slope of labrum.) B. Transverse view in flexion. Note the U formed by
the metaphysis and acetabulum. (m = metaphysis; h = head of femur;
i = ischium.)

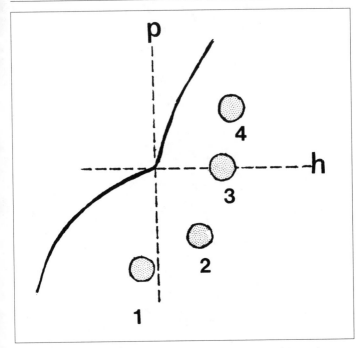

Fig. 2-4. Tonnis grades 1–4 of hip dislocation. (p = Perkins' line; h = Hilgenreiner's line.)

    G. Management of hip dysplasia. Figure 2-7 shows a general algorithm for management of dysplasia. Guidelines given are approximate and must be modified based on individual factors.

Bibliography

Boeree NR, Clarke NMP. Ultrasound imaging and secondary screening for congenital dislocation of the hip. *J Bone Joint Surg [Br]* 76:525, 1994.

Harke HT, Kumar JS. Current concepts review: The role of ultrasound in the diagnosis and management of congenital dislocation of the hip. *J Bone Joint Surg [Am]* 73:622, 1991.

Weinstein SL. Developmental Dysplasia of the Hip. In RT Morrissey (ed), *Pediatric Orthopaedics* (4th ed). Philadelphia: Lippincott, 1996.

II. Legg-Calvé-Perthes disease (Perthes disease)
    A. Principles. Legg-Calvé-Perthes disease (idiopathic avascular necrosis of the femoral head) is most commonly seen in children aged 4–10. Ten percent of patients develop

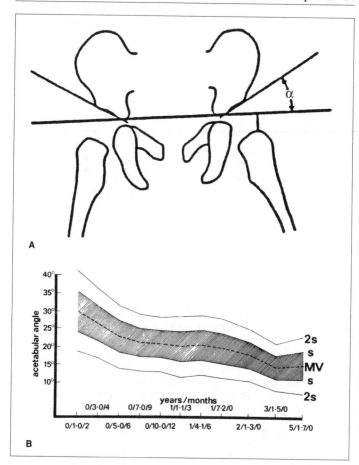

Fig. 2-5. A. Acetabular index measurement. (alpha = acetabular roof
line.) B. Normal values of the acetabular index by age (girls). (s = 1
standard deviation; 2s = 2 standard deviations; MV = mean value.)
(Reproduced with permission from D Tonnis. Normal values of the hip
joint for evaluation of x-rays. *Clin Orthop* 119:39, 1976.)

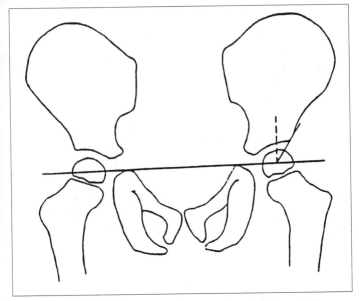

Fig. 2-6. Center edge angle of Wiberg. (Reproduced with permission from D Tonnis. Normal values of the hip joint for evaluation of x-rays. *Clin Orthop* 119:39, 1976.)

bilateral involvement, but this involvement almost always occurs at different times (asynchronous). Synchronous involvement should suggest the possibility of other causes.

B. Symptoms
   1. Minimal or no history of trauma
   2. Stiffness
   3. Intermittent, mild pain or no pain
C. Signs
   1. Mild Trendelenburg gait
   2. No spasm with gentle motion
   3. Limitation of extremes of motion, especially abduction and internal rotation
D. Radiographic findings
   1. Chronologic sequence
      a. Initially may appear normal
      b. Failure of nucleus to grow compared to opposite side
      c. Subchondral "crescent" sign, best seen on lateral view, present in one-third of cases. It is a lucent arc central to subchondral bone respresenting a compression fracture.
      d. Fragmentation of nucleus with resorption
      e. Epiphyseal extrusion
      f. Physeal and metaphyseal osteolysis and irregularity
      g. Reossification and variable remodeling
      h. Usually slight loss of epiphyseal and neck height at final appearance

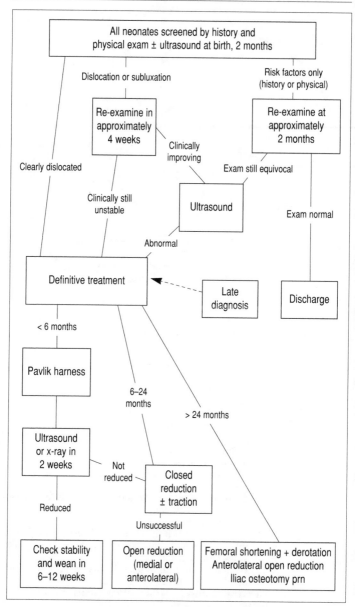

Fig. 2-7. General algorithm for management of pediatric hip dysplasia.

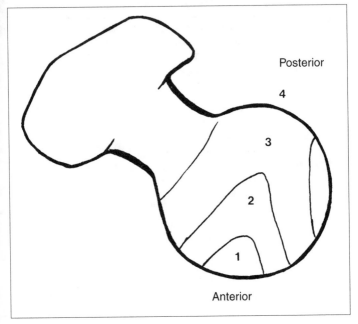

Fig. 2-8. Catterall classification of Perthes disease (transverse view).

2. **Staging**
   a. **Catterall classification** (Fig. 2-8)
      (1) 1: Central anterior involvement of head only
      (2) 2: Greater central head involvement, but intact medial and lateral column
      (3) 3: Lateral three-fourths of femoral head involved only with intact medial column; metaphyseal reaction
      (4) 4: Whole-head involvement, with metaphyseal reaction and remodeling of epiphysis
   b. **Salter classification**
      (1) A: Less than half of femoral head involved; intact lateral pillar (corresponds to Catterall stages 1 and 2)
      (2) B: More than half of head involved; lateral pillar involved (Catterall stages 3 and 4)
   c. **Herring lateral pillar classification.** Predicts flattening during healing (Fig. 2-9).
      (1) A: Lateral pillar intact without radiographic change (Fig. 2-9A)
      (2) B: Lateral pillar collapsed, but height still 50% or more of orginal height (Fig. 2-9B)
      (3) C: Lateral pillar collapsed to less than 50% of the original height (Fig. 2-9C)

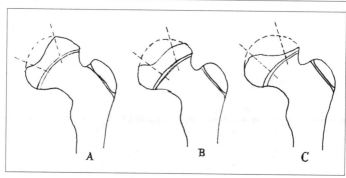

Fig. 2-9. Herring lateral pillar classification of Perthes disease from A to C for increasing severity. (Originally described in JA Herring, et al. Evolution of the femoral head deformity during the healing phases of Legg-Calvé-Perthes Disease.)

3. Prognostic signs

    a. Head-at-risk signs of Catterall

        (1) Lateral calcification

        (2) Lateral subluxation

        (3) Gage sign: lucency proximal and distal to lateral physis

        (4) Metaphyseal reaction

        (5) Horizontal physis (meaning limb is adducted)

    b. Epiphyseal extrusion (Fig. 2-10) greater than 20% carries poor long-term prognosis.

    c. Mose sphericity: Deviation of head periphery from a perfect sphere by more than 3 mm on anteroposterior and lateral radiograph carries a poor long-term prognosis.

    d. Stulberg rating (at healing) assesses femoral head sphericity and its congruency with the acetabulum. Stulberg's five stages have been correlated with long-term outcome (Fig. 2-11).

  4. Arthrogram or MRI is not routinely indicated but may be helpful in some cases.

E. Differential diagnosis

  1. Hypothyroidism

  2. Multiple epiphyseal dysplasia

  3. Spondyloepiphyseal dysplasia

  4. Storage disorder (Gaucher's disease, mucopolysaccharidoses)

  5. Avascular necrosis (AVN) following trauma, steroids, sickle cell infarct, treatment for DDH

F. Treatment

  1. There is no consensus on a protocol, but while many hips have a poor long-term natural outcome, some hips appear to be helped by treatment. **Containment** is indicated if several of the following features are present:

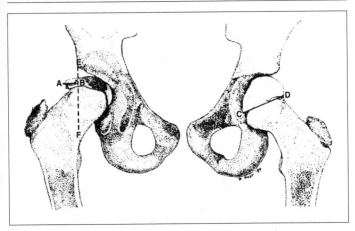

Fig. 2-10. Measurement of epiphyseal extrusion = AB/CD. (A,B = width of involved epiphysis lateral to Perkins' line; C,D = medial and lateral borders of normal epiphysis; E,F = Perkins' line.) (Reproduced with permission from NE Greene. Epiphyseal extrusion as a prognostic index in Legg-Calve-Perthes disease. *J Bone Joint Surg [Am]* 63:900, 1981.)

        a. Head involvement greater than 50% (Caterall 3–4, Salter B, Herring B or C)
        b. Age greater than 6 years
        c. Persistent stiffness
        d. Collapse or extrusion not established yet
    2. Containment options
        a. Abduction brace or Petrie casts
        b. Femoral varus osteotomy
        c. Iliac rotational osteotomy or augmentation
        d. Combination of *b* and *c* (above)
    3. Late options
        a. Epiphysiodesis for leg length inequality greater than 2 cm
        b. Valgus osteotomy for symptomatic hinge abduction
        c. Trochanteric transfer for persistent abductor weakness

Bibliography

Wenger DR, Ward WT, Herring JA. Current concepts review: Legg Calvé Perthes disease. *J Bone Joint Surg [Am]* 73:778, 1991.

III. Slipped capital femoral epiphysis
    A. Background
        1. Incidence: 1–10 per 100,000
            a. Higher in males than females and higher in African-Americans
            b. Twenty percent have bilateral involvement at presentation; 20% become bilateral later

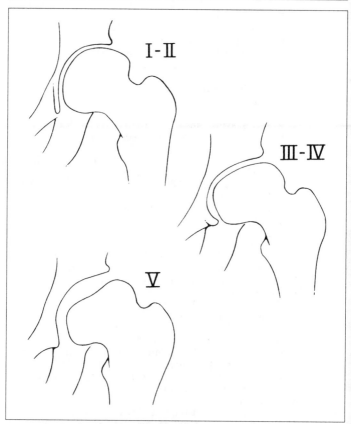

Fig. 2-11. Stulberg rating of outcome of healed Perthes disease. Stages I and II are spherical and congruent and carry a low likelihood of degenerative joint disease. Stages III and IV are aspheric and congruous and carry a risk of degenerative joint disease by middle age. Stage V is aspheric and incongruous and carries a risk of degenerative joint disease before 50. (Reproduced with permission from SD Stulberg. The natural history of Legg-Perthes disease. *J Bone Joint Surg [Am]* 63:1095, 1981.)

    2. Etiologic factors

      a. Obesity

      b. Mild or severe trauma

      c. Endocrinologic factors: hypothyroidism, hypogo-nadism, rickets, renal failure

      d. Down syndrome

      e. Positive family history

B. Classification

    1. Chronologic

      a. Acute: symptoms of less than 3 weeks' duration

      b. Chronic: symptoms for 3 weeks or more

    2. Severity

      a. "Pre-slip": symptoms present in patient at risk, but no observable slip; MRI may be positive.

      b. Grade I: less than 33% slip of epiphysis on metaphysis

      c. Grade II: 33–50% slip

      d. Grade III: more than 50% slip

C. Clinical presentation

    1. Age 9–14

    2. Antalgic limp

    3. Pain in the thigh, knee, or hip

    4. Leg externally rotated during gait and at rest

    5. Internal rotation less in flexion than extension

D. Radiography

    1. Slip best seen on lateral view

    2. Anteroposterior view

      a. Physeal widening and irregularity

      b. Decreased epiphyseal height

      c. Klein's line (line on lateral femoral neck) transects less than 20% of epiphysis in child over age 10.

      d. Chondrolysis (joint space narrowing) may be seen before treatment (rare).

E. Treatment

    1. Immediate weight relief (bed rest)

    2. For acute slip, traction for comfort or reduction if severe (optional)

    3. Fixation in situ:

      a. Screw

        (1) Single, centrally placed within physis

        (2) Two screws may be used if first is imperfect or if slip is severe or unstable.

      b. Bone graft epiphysiodesis (less commonly used)

    4. Realignment. The main indication for realignment is a patient who is unsatisfied with limb deformity resulting from slip; not commonly needed.

      a. Cuneiform osteotomy just below physis

      b. Base-of-neck osteotomy; some series show high rate of AVN

      c. Subtrochanteric valgus-flexion-derotation osteotomy

    5. Prophylactic contralateral pinning may be indicated in a patient in whom diagnosis of late contralateral slipped capital femoral epiphysis may be missed due to impaired communication or follow-up.

F. Complications

    1. Chondrolysis (5%) usually improves with time and therapy

2. Avascular necrosis
   a. Greater in acute or unstable slips
   b. May be focal or complete
   c. Some healing possible

Bibliography

Crawford AH. Current concepts review—Slipped capital femoral epiphysis. *J Bone Joint Surg [Am]* 70:1422, 1988.

IV. Developmental coxa vara
   A. Definition. Developmental coxa vara is a varus deformity of the femoral neck that is usually progressive. Incidence is 1 in 25,000. Thirty percent of cases are bilateral.
   B. Radiographic features
   1. Femoral neck shortened and bent inward (varus)
   2. Inverted-Y appearance of physis
   3. Triangular fragment on inferior femoral neck
   4. Decreased femoral anteversion
   5. Mild acetabular dysplasia
   C. Signs and symptoms
   1. Progressive gait deterioration, due to abductor weakness and leg length inequality
   2. Occasional hip pain
   3. Length inequality, if unilateral, usually less than 2.5 cm
   D. Differential diagnosis
   1. Cleidocranial dysplasia
   2. Metaphyseal dysplasia
   3. Morquio's syndrome
   E. Treatment
   1. If Hilgenreiner-epiphyseal angle is less than 45 degrees, observe (Fig. 2-12).
   2. If Hilgenreiner-epiphyseal angle exceeds 45 degrees and deformity is progressive and symptomatic, or if Hilgenreiner-epiphyseal angle exceeds 60 degrees at diagnosis, perform valgus derotation osteotomy.

Bibliography

Weinstein JN, Kuo KN, Millar EA. Congenital coxa vara. A retrospective review. *J Pediatr Orthop* 4:70, 1984.

V. Proximal focal femoral deficiency
   A. Definition. Proximal focal femoral deficiency describes the group of congenital femoral anomalies that include a temporary or permanent discontinuity in the proximal femur.
   B. Classification. The most commonly used system is the Aitken classification (Fig. 2-13):
   1. A: The femur is continuous but appears discontinuous early due to incomplete ossification of cartilage.
   2. B: The varus or shortening of the proximal segment is more extreme, but most cases ossify later.

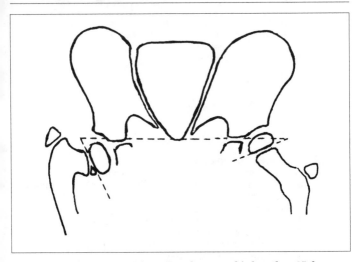

Fig. 2-12. Hilgenreiner-epiphyseal angle; normal is less than 25 degrees (left hip). Note the inverted-Y appearance of physis on involved right hip. (Reproduced with permission from JN Weinstein. Congenital coxa vara. A retrospective review. *J Pediatr Orthop* 4:70, 1984.)

    3. C: The acetabulum is small and the femoral head is absent.
    4. D: Both the femoral head and the acetabulum are absent.
        There are other classification systems, such as those of Kalamchi and Pappas, but they are less widely used.

C. Characteristics
    1. Fifteen percent are bilateral (most are Aitken type D).
    2. Over 50% of patients with proximal focal femoral deficiency have other lower extremity anomalies, most commonly fibular hemimelia.
    3. Growth retardation is a constant proportion of the normal limb.

D. Problems
    1. Limb length inequality (if unilateral).
    2. Pelvic-femoral instability
    3. Malrotation of lower extremity (flexion-abduction-external rotation)
    4. Proximal muscle weakness

E. Treatment
    1. Bilateral
        a. Patients walk well without prostheses if feet are normal.
        b. Nonfunctional feet may need revision.
        c. Extension prostheses may be used when desired to increase height.
    2. Unilateral
        a. Hip abnormalities: Perform valgus osteotomy for types A and B; for type D, consider femoropelvic arthrodesis rather than containment of thigh segment in a prosthesis.

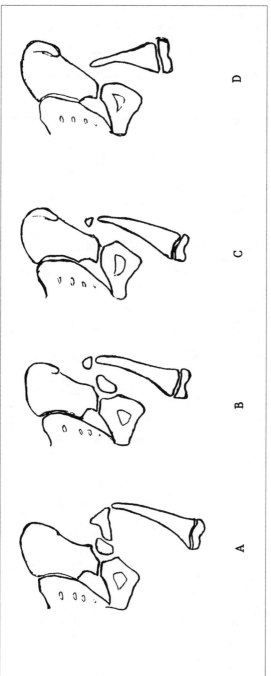

Fig. 2-13. Proximal focal femoral deficiency: Aitken classification (A–D).

    b. Knee: Offer rotationplasty if foot and ankle are strong and positioned distal to the contralateral knee. Syme's amputation is another option, combined with fusion of anatomic knee to increase lever arm.

    c. Foot: Prosthesis equalizes length and provides a functional foot.

Bibliography

Aitken GT. Proximal femoral focal deficiency: Definition, classification and management. *Proc Natl Acad Sci USA* 1734:1, 1969.

Kalamchi A, Cowell HR, Kim KI. Congenital deficiency of the femur. *J Pediatr Orthop* 5:129, 1985.

Pappas AM. Congenital abnormalities of the femur and related lower extremity malformations. *J Pediatr Orthop* 3:45, 1983.

VI. Tibia vara
  A. Definition. Tibia vara (also known as Blount disease) is a focal varus deformity of the proximal tibia due to mechanical overload of the medial growth plate causing disordered growth. It may occur in infantile, juvenile, or adolescent age groups.
  B. Clinical presentation (Table 2-1)
  C. Radiographic features
    1. Normal alignment of the lower extremity is shown in Figure 1-33.
    2. In infantile tibia vara, changes involve physeal depression with lucency and beaking of the corresponding metaphysis and epiphysis. These changes have been staged by Langenskjold (Fig. 2-14), but interobserver correlation is poor.
    3. Infants under age 2 have inadequate ossification to designate Langenskjold stages. As an alternate means of early diagnosis, the metaphyseal-diaphyseal angle

Table 2-1. Comparison of tibia vara types (by age)

	Infantile	Juvenile	Adolescent
Age (yrs)	0–3	3–10	11 and older
Painful	No	No	Usually
Site of varus	Proximal tibia only; medial plateau may be tilted or depressed.	—	Distal femur and proximal tibia
Treatment	Femur often in valgus; observe or brace; perform tibial osteotomy if not better by age 4.	—	Osteotomy of tibia with or without femur as indicated

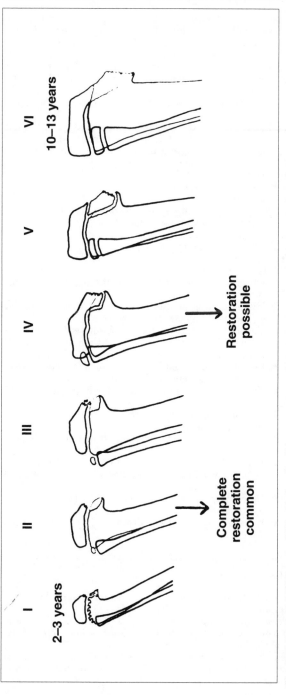

Fig. 2-14. Langenskjold stages I–VI of infantile tibia vara. (Reproduced with permission from A Langenskjold. Tibia vara. *Acta Chirurg Scand* 103:9, 1952.)

should be drawn. A line through medial and lateral beaks of the metaphysis forms an angle with the diaphysis (Fig. 2-15). An angle of greater than 11–16 degrees is good evidence for Blount disease.

4. Medial physeal slope greater than 60 degrees may predict recurrent bowing after osteotomy (Fig. 2-16). It is measured as the angle between the most straight portions of the medial and lateral segments of the physis.

5. Medial plateau depression is measured as the angle between the medial and lateral portions of the tibial plateau. A value greater than 30 degrees may be seen in neglected infantile tibia vara (Fig. 2-17).

D. Differential diagnosis

1. Rickets (many types)
2. Achondroplasia
3. Metaphyseal chondrodysplasia (Schmidt type)
4. Trauma or infection of medial physis
5. Physiologic bowing
6. Focal fibrocartilaginous dysplasia

E. Treatment

1. Infantile tibia vara
   a. Observe or brace (day vs. night according to the physician's preference).
   b. Valgus derotation tibial osteotomy if not better by age 4 or if Langenskjold stage IV.
   c. Consider tomograms for bar if physis is narrow or medial physeal slope is greater than 60 degrees. If bar is found, resect it or close lateral side of physis.
   d. Consider tibial plateau elevation if medial plateau depression exceeds 25 degrees.
   e. Correct femoral valgus deformity if greater than 10 degrees.
   f. Equalize leg lengths as needed.
2. Adolescent tibia vara
   a. Correct if deformity exceeds 10 degrees or if pain persists.
   b. Lateral hemiepiphysiodesis is an option if deformity is not severe and patient has 2 or more years of growth remaining.
   c. Osteotomy of proximal tibia and distal femur as appropriate.
   d. Equalize leg lengths if discrepancy is greater than 2.5 cm.

Bibliography

Greene WB. Infantile tibia vara. Instructional course lecture. *J Bone Joint Surg [Am]* 75:130, 1993.

Henderson RC, Kemp GJ, Greene WB. Adolescent tibia vara: Alternatives for treatment. *J Bone Joint Surg [Am]* 74:342,1992.

Schoenecker PL, Johnston R, Rich MM et al. Elevation of the medial plateau of the tibia in the treatment of Blount disease. *J Bone Joint Surg [Am]* 74:351, 1992.

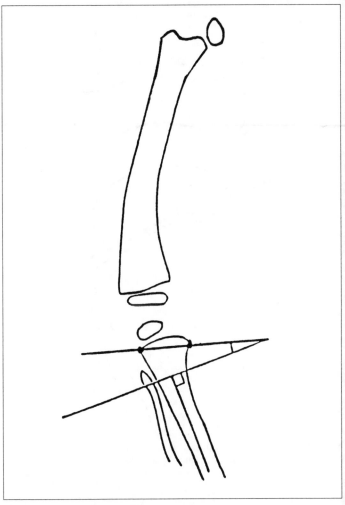

Fig. 2-15. The metaphyseal-diaphyseal angle; there is a high diagnostic likelihood of tibia vara if the angle is greater than 11–16 degrees.

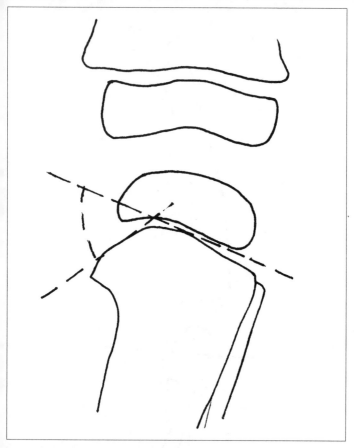

Fig. 2-16. The medial physeal slope is used to predict the risk of recurrent deformity. Values greater than 60 degrees indicate increased risk.

VII. Other angular deformities about the knee

A. Evaluation. Angular deformities may occur as a result of trauma or metabolic disorders, or they may be idiopathic. If deviation from normal alignment is greater than 10 degrees, correction may be indicated in some cases.

B. Treatment. Treatment may be done by osteotomy and internal or external fixation or by hemiepiphysiodesis. The goal is to restore a horizontal joint line, physiologic angulation (see Chap. 1, Fig. 1-33), and near-equal limb lengths.

Hemiepiphysiodesis may be the simplest method of correction for some patients. The theory is illustrated in Figure 2-18A. Prerequisites include (1) predictable growth pattern, (2) sufficient growth remaining to correct defect, and (3) limb lengths close to equal.

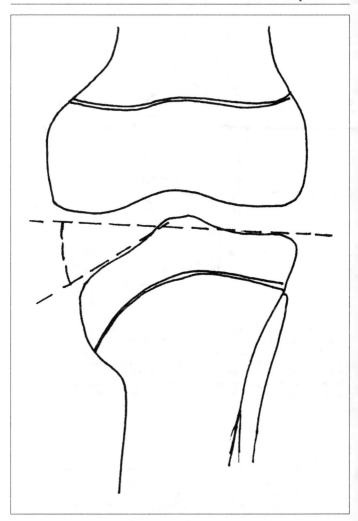

Fig. 2-17. Medial plateau depression is unique to infantile tibia vara; if greater than 30 degrees, the medial side may need to be selectively elevated.

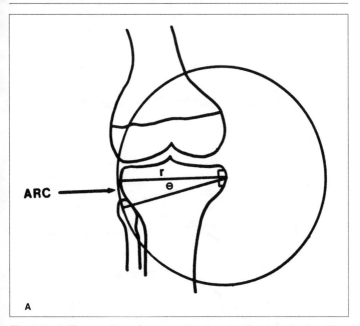

Fig. 2-18. A. Theory of angular correction by asymmetric tethering. The angle of deformity (θ) may be represented by the arc of a circle having a radius (r). This arc also approximates the amount of semilateral growth inhibition required to correct the deformity. **B.** Angular correction is calculated from metaphyseal width and growth remaining. (Reproduced with permission from JR Bowen. Hemiepiphysiodesis to correct angular deformity of the knee. *Clin Orthop* 198:185, 1985.)

   C. Planning (Fig. 2-18B)
      1. Locate site of angular deformity—distal femur, proximal tibia, or both—and measure its degree.
      2. Determine relative length (compared to mean standard deviation for age) of the patient's femur or tibia using Figure 1-17 in Chapter 1.
      3. Using the width of the physis and the desired degree of correction, draw a horizontal line on the figure.
      4. Draw a dot at the intersection of this horizontal line with the patient's tibial or femoral percentile.
      5. A vertical line from this point downward indicates the age at which hemiepiphysiodesis should be performed.

Bibliography

Bowen JR, Leahy LJ, Zhang Z, MacEwen GD. Hemiepiphysiodesis to correct angular deformity about the knee. *Clin Orthop* 198:184, 1985.

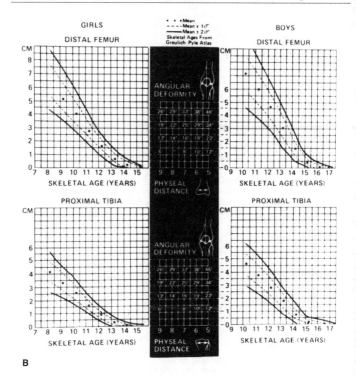

GIRLS

DISTAL FEMUR

BOYS

DISTAL FEMUR

PROXIMAL TIBIA

PROXIMAL TIBIA

ANGULAR
DEFORMITY

PHYSEAL
DISTANCE

• • • Mean
- - - - Mean ± 1σ
——— Mean ± 2σ
Skeletal Ages From
Greulich Pyle Atlas

B

Fig. 2-18. *(continued)*

VIII. Patellofemoral disorders

   A. Principles. Patellofemoral disorders are common in children, especially in adolescents. A standardized approach aids in diagnosis. History should include duration of symptoms, recent changes in activity, and factors that bring about the pain.

   B. Physical examination. The physical examination should be systematic.

     1. Ask the patient to point to the location of pain.
     2. Test for pain on compression of patella.
     3. Perform apprehension test.
     4. Check for effusion.
     5. Note any retinacular tightness (reverse tilt).
     6. Measure tibial and femoral rotational alignment.
     7. Assess ligament and meniscal integrity.
     8. Measure valgus.
     9. Examine active tracking.
     10. Observe gait.

   C. Differential diagnosis. The following disorders may produce symptoms in the patellofemoral region:

     1. Symptomatic plica syndrome
     2. Saphenous nerve entrapment

   3. Fat pad impingement
   4. Patellar osteochondritis
   5. Iliotibial band syndrome
   6. Patellar malalignment
   7. Patellar subluxation
   8. Combination of one or more of the above, with or without arthrosis
 D. Radiographic evaluation. X-rays are not needed on initial evaluation of all cases. If the problem is recalcitrant, however, the following studies may help.
   1. Merchant view: a "sunrise" view taken at 30–45 degrees of knee flexion (Fig. 2-19A). From this, the **sulcus angle**, which should be greater than –17 degrees (Fig. 2-19B), can be measured.
   2. The lateral view shows the Insall ratio, which is the length of the patellar tendon divided by the length of the patella (Fig. 2-20). The mean for the population is 1.0, and the upper limit of normal is 1.2. **Patella alta** is defined as an Insall ratio (length of tendon divided by length of patella) greater than 1.2.
   3. CT may be helpful to assess **patellar tilt**. The CT scan should be performed with the knee in 20 degrees flexion (Fig. 2-21). Normal patellar tilt is greater than 8 degrees.
 E. Treatment. Treatment of routine patellofemoral malalignment should start with conservative measures. These may include the following:
   1. Stretching of retinaculum, iliotibial (IT) band, quadriceps, and hamstrings.
   2. Strengthening of quadriceps: Use low resistance, high repetition with the knee not flexed over 45 degrees to minimize force on the patellar cartilage.
   3. Nonsteroidal anti-inflammatory drugs.
   4. Orthotics to decrease pronation of the foot with its resultant external tibial torsion.
   5. Elastic brace or patellar taping.
   6. In the rare case resistant to treatments 1–5, if significant limitations persist, surgical correction may be offered. This may include one or more of the following options:
     a. Lateral release (for patellar tilt)
     b. Tibial tubercle transfer with or without vastus medialis obliquus (VMO) advancement (for subluxation)
     c. Limited debridement (for severe cartilage surface degeneration)

IX. Clubfoot
 A. Etiology. Talipes equinovarus (clubfoot) can be unilateral or bilateral with approximately equal frequency. Although most cases are idiopathic, other causes or associations should be considered:
   1. Neurogenic: spinal dysraphism, tethered cord, arthrogryposis
   2. Connective tissue disorders: Larsen's syndrome, diastrophic dwarfism
   3. Mechanical: oligohydramnios, congenital constriction bands

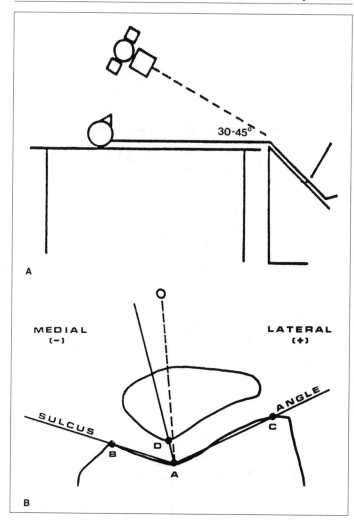

Fig. 2-19. A. Merchant view, a sunrise view with knee flexed 30–45 degrees. B. Interpretation: Sulcus angle should be at least –17 degrees. (AO is the bisector of the angle; ABC is drawn from the femoral trochlear.) (Reproduced with permission from AC Merchant. Roentgenographic analyses of patellofemoral congruence. *J Bone Joint Surg [Am]* 56:1395, 1974.)

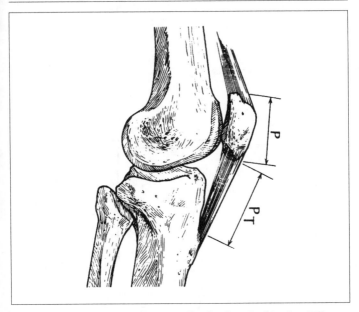

Fig. 2-20. Insall ratio to evaluate patella alta: length of tendon (PT) divided by length of patella (P). Patella alta is defined as an Insall ratio greater than 1.2. (Reproduced with permission from JN Insall. Chondromalacia patellae: A prospective study. *J Bone Joint Surg [Am]* 58:1, 1976.)

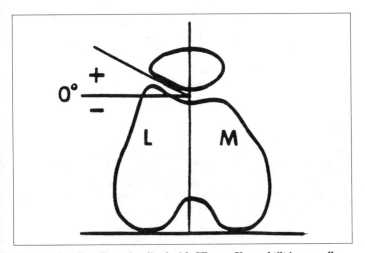

Fig. 2-21. Patellar tilt as visualized with CT scan. Upward tilt is normally greater than 8 degrees. (L = lateral; M = medial angle of tilt drawn between the lateral patellar facet and the posterior femoral condylar line or a line parallel to it.) (Reproduced with permission from SF Schutzer, GR Ramsby, JP Fulkerson. The evaluation of patellofemoral pain using computerized tomography. A preliminary study. *Clin Orthop* 204:286, 1986.)

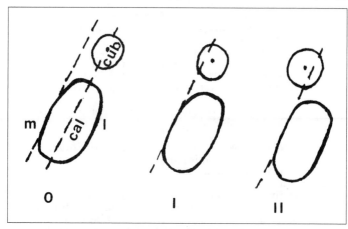

Fig. 2-22. Calcaneocuboid relationship: The centers of the calcaneus (cal) and the cuboid (cub) are located, and the calcaneus is divided into halves. Grade 0: the center of the cuboid is aligned with the midline of the calcaneus; grade I: the center of the cuboid is medial to the midline; grade II: the cuboid is medial to the cortex of the calcaneus. (m = medial; l = lateral.)

   4. Other: Freeman-Sheldon syndrome, Pierre Robin syndrome, tibial hemimelia
  B. **Physical findings.** One or more of these findings may be present. The foot may be given a score from 1 to 10 if each positive finding is awarded 1 point.
   1. Medial or posterior crease
   2. Curved lateral border
   3. Calf atrophy
   4. External rotation of lateral malleolus
   5. Talipes cavus
   6. Talipes equinus
   7. Hindfoot stiffness (calcaneus fixed to fibula)
   8. Midfoot stiffness
   9. Forefoot supination
   10. Navicular bone fixed to medial malleolus
  C. **Radiographic features**
   1. Radiographs are useful primarily when surgery is indicated or in postsurgical follow-up. Anteroposterior and lateral films should be taken with the foot plantigrade. Normal values for anteroposterior and lateral talocalcaneal angles are given in Figures 1-39A and B in Chapter 1. Talipes equinovarus is associated with increasing parallelism of the talus and calcaneus.
   2. The calcaneocuboid relationship can be graded 0, I, or II (Fig. 2-22), as follows: The centers of the calcaneus and the cuboid are located and the calcaneus divided in half. If the center of the cuboid aligns with the midline of the calcaneus, the calcaneocuboid relationship is grade 0. Grade I is defined as the center of cuboid lying medial to the midline, and grade II as the cuboid lying medial to the

cortex of the calcaneus. A calcaneocuboid release should be included in operative treatment of grade II feet.

D. Treatment
   1. Manipulation and cast. If treatment is successful, correction may need to be held with splints or straight-last shoes and a Denis Browne splint.
   2. Operative correction, depending on severity, may include:
      a. Lengthening of heel cord and posterior tibialis
      b. Posteromedial capsulotomies
      c. Complete subtalar release
      d. Calcaneocuboid release if grade II calcaneocuboid malalignment is present
      e. Lateral column shortening

X. Tarsal coalition
   A. Definition. Tarsal coalition is a fibrous, cartilaginous, or bony connection of two or more tarsal bones. It is present in about 3% of the population and is bilateral in half of these. Calcaneonavicular (CN) and talocalcaneal (TC) bars are the two most common types.

   B. Signs and symptoms
      1. Foot or ankle pain and stiffness occurs at about ages 8–12 for calcaneonavicular bar, ages 12–16 for talocalcaneal bar.
      2. Limitation of subtalar movement is greater with talocalcaneal coalition than with calcaneonavicular bar.
      3. Pes planus (variable).
      4. Peroneal guarding or "spasm."

   C. Radiographs
      1. Oblique view of the midfoot is diagnostic for CN bar with narrowing, irregularity, or fusion of the space between the two bones.
      2. Lateral view shows pointed projection of calcaneus, or "anteater nose," in TC coalition.
      3. Harris view shows obliquity and sclerosis of the sustentaculum in TC coalition and may show fusion across the middle facet. This view is taken with the patient standing on the cassette, knees and ankles flexed, and the beam angled down 35–45 degrees from posterior to anterior.
      4. CT scan is the definitive study for a TC coalition. The plane of the tomograms should be the coronal plane of the foot with knees flexed and the sole flat on gantry.
      5. CN and TC coalitions may coexist.

   D. Treatment
      1. If discovered incidentally and asymptomatic, observe
      2. Orthotic, if the foot is not rigid
      3. Walking cast for 3–6 weeks
      4. Bar resection (A) if conservative treatment fails for TC bar less than 50% with no degenerative changes or (B) for CN bar of any size
      5. Arthrodesis of appropriate joints

XI. Idiopathic scoliosis
   A. Background. Idiopathic scoliosis is the most common pediatric spinal deformity. It is transmittted as an autosomal dominant condition with incomplete penetrance. The

Table 2-2. Tanner stages

Stage	Boys	Girls
I	Childhood genitalia	Elevation of papilla
II	Scrotum and testes enlarged	Breast bud (breast and papilla)
III	Enlargement of penis	Further enlargement of breast and areola
IV	Development of glands, darkening of scrotum	Projection of areola and papilla
V	Adult size and hair pattern	Mature stage: projection of papilla only

initial evaluation should rule out other causes and determine maturity, curve size, type, and appropriate treatment.

B. History
1. How curve was discovered
2. Presence or absence of significant pain
3. Family history
4. Menarchal status
5. Prior medical and surgical history

C. Physical examination
1. Record height and weight.
2. Brief general examination of trunk and extremities for cutaneous lesions, congenital malformation, connective tissue disorder, or atrophy
3. Screen for lower limb length inequality
4. Neurologic examination
   a. Strength and reflexes in all extremities
   b. Abdominal reflex testing
   c. Straight-leg raising test
5. Estimate physical maturity (direct examination unnecessary unless critical treatment decision is pending) (Table 2-2).
6. Assess curve pattern.
   a. Shoulder elevation
   b. Trunk balance C7–S1, in coronal and sagittal planes
   c. Curve level
   d. Intrinsic pelvic deformity
   e. Kyphosis and lordosis
   f. Scoliosis screening: forward-bend test (Fig. 2-23)
      (1) Have patient stand with feet together, knees straight, and palms together. Check shoulders and pelvis for obliquity, and equalize leg lengths with blocks if necessary. Observe sagittal profile for focal kyphosis.
      (2) Have patient bend slowly **all** the way over (see Fig. 2-23D).
      (3) Check thoracic spine.
      (4) Check lumbar spine (Fig. 2-24).
      (5) Perform scoliometer measurement of trunk asymmetry. The scoliometer measures the angle of trunk rotation. This is roughly correlated with

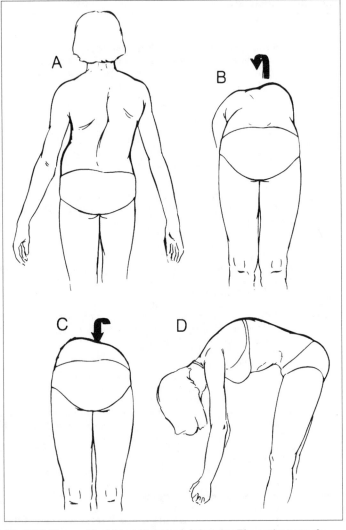

Fig. 2-23. Forward-bend test for spinal deformity. The patient stands with feet together and knees straight (A) and slowly bends forward to touch the toes (arrows). The spine is observed continuously from early bend (B) to late bend (C), as well as from the lateral position (D).

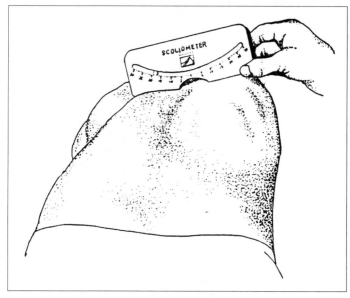

Fig. 2-24. Technique of scoliometer measurement. (Reproduced with permission from WP Bunnell. An objective criterion for scoliosis screening. *J Bone Joint Surg [Am]* **66:1383, 1984.)**

the Cobb angle (Fig. 2-25). A scoliometer reading of 5 degrees or less is 99% sensitive and 97% specific for curves less than a 20-degree Cobb angle. The mean Cobb measurement for 5-degree curves by scoliometer is 11 degrees. The scoliometer is adequately sensitive for scoliosis screening.

D. Differential diagnosis (in absence of overt vertebral malformations)

    1. Genetic or connective tissue disorders

        a. Marfan syndrome

        b. Ehlers-Danlos syndrome

        c. Neurofibromatosis

        d. Prader-Willi syndrome

        e. Stickler syndrome

        f. Many others

    2. Neurologic disease

        a. Syringomyelia

        b. Brain stem or cord tumor

        c. Friedreich's ataxia

        d. Charcot-Marie-Tooth disease

        e. Poliomyelitis

        f. Thoracic level paralysis or lack of coordination of any cause

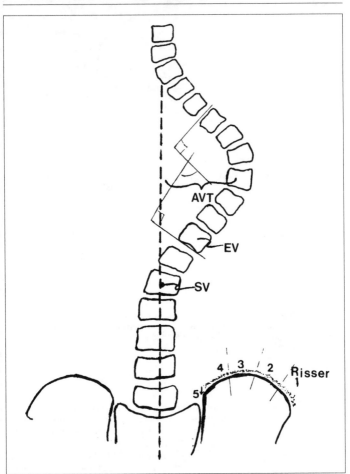

Fig. 2-25. Radiographic assessment of spinal curvature. The Cobb angle is the most commonly accepted method for quantifying spinal curves. It is the angle between the upper and lower end vertebrae (EV) in the curve. Risser sign reflects maturation of the ilium. Risser 0 (no secondary ossification center) indicates significant spinal growth potential. Risser 5 (fused epiphyses) correlates roughly with skeletal maturity and helps predict the end of skeletal growth, but the Risser sign should not be used in isolation. The stable vertebra (SV) is the lowest vertebra bisected by a vertical line from the center of the sacrum. The apical vertebral translation (AVT) is measured with respect to the center sacral line.

3. Neoplastic and other conditions
   a. Tethered cord or occult dysraphism
   b. Osteoid osteoma
   c. Osteoblastoma
   d. Postradiation
   e. Spinal cord tumor

E. **Radiographic assessment**
   1. A radiograph should be taken if the physical examination indicates that a curve may require treatment. Posteroanterior technique minimizes dose to gonads and breasts but gives slightly less detail. A lateral film should be ordered only if specifically needed for evaluation of pain or deformity.
   2. Radiographs should be analyzed for the presence of other anomalies, such as congenital malformation, vertebral erosion, or pedicle widening or thinning. The curve magnitude may be described by the Cobb measurement, the direction of convexity, and the vertebral levels involved. The interobserver Cobb measurement error is 6 degrees for idiopathic scoliosis and more than 10 degrees for congenital scoliosis. Skeletal maturity may be estimated by the Risser sign, but this should be correlated with physical examination (Tanner stage) and bone age if needed.
   3. Rotation in the adolescent may be estimated by the method of Nash and Moe (Fig. 2-26), by CT scan, or by the Perdriolle method.
   4. Rotation may be estimated in the infantile or juvenile patient using the rib-vertebral angle difference of Mehta (Fig. 2-27).
   5. Curve types are named for level of the apex:
      a. Thoracolumbar curves have an apex at T11–L1. Thoracic curves have an apex above this level; lumbar curves have an apex below this level.
      b. King has classified thoracic curves into five types (Fig. 2-28).

         I   True double major curves of equal magnitude and flexibility
         II False double major curves; lumbar curve is smaller and more flexible with less prominence
         III Thoracic curve only; lumbar curve does not cross middle
         IV Long thoracic curve; returns to midline at L4
         V   Double thoracic curve

G. **Treatment algorithm for idiopathic scoliosis.** This algorithm serves as an overview of scoliosis management (Fig. 2-29). It represents mainstream thought on the subject, but each case must be managed individually.

Bibliography

Bunnell WP. Outcome of spinal screening. *Spine* 18:1572, 1993.
Bunnell WP. An objective criterion for scoliosis screening. *J Bone Joint Surg [Am]* 66:1381, 1984.

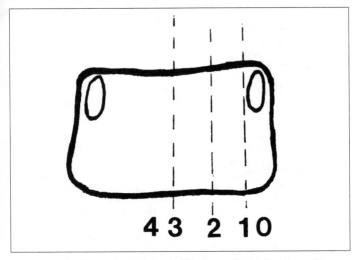

Fig. 2-26. Rotation may be estimated by the method of Nash and Moe, according to the location of the pedicle on the convex side. The midpoint of the vertebra is defined, and the half on the convex side is divided into thirds. The status of the convex pedicle with respect to these landmarks is noted as shown (1–4).

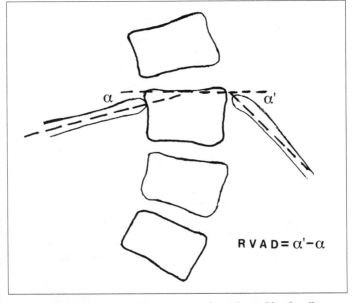

Fig. 2-27. Rotation in infantile curves may be estimated by the rib vertebral angle difference (RVAD) of Mehta. This is the difference between the angles (α and α') formed by the two ribs versus the end plate of the apical vertebra.

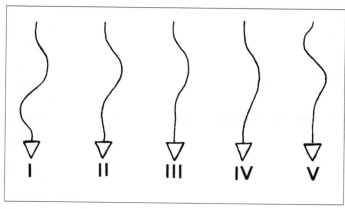

Fig. 2-28. The King classification of thoracic curve types.

King HA. The section of fusion levels in thoracic idiopathic scoliosis. *J Bone Joint Surg [Am]* 65:1302, 1983.

Mehta MH. The rib-vertebral angle in the early diagnosis between resolving and progressive infantile scoliosis. *J Bone Joint Surg [Br]* 54:230, 1972.

Nash CL Jr, Moe JH. A study of vertebral rotation. *J Bone Joint Surg [Am]* 51:223, 1969.

XII. Back pain in children

  A. Significance. Although disabling back pain in children is rare, back pain of some degree is experienced by over 30% of children.

    1. History

      a. Mechanism of onset

      b. Duration

      c. Severity (1–10)

      d. Interference with school, play, or sports

    2. Physical examination

      a. Neurologic examination

      b. Spinal range of motion

      c. Location of pain

      d. Straight-leg raising test

  B. Differential diagnosis

    1. Developmental disorders

      a. Spondylolysis (most common)

      b. Scheuermann's kyphosis (second most common)

      c. Tethered cord

    2. Trauma

      a. Herniated nucleus pulposus or end plate

      b. Musculoligamentous strain

      c. Fracture

    3. Infectious disease

      a. Discitis

      b. Osteomyelitis

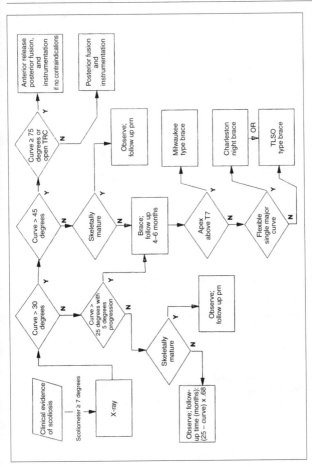

Fig. 2-29. Idiopathic scoliosis treatment algorithm. (TRC = triradiate cartilage; TLSO = thoracolumbosacral orthosis.) (Reproduced with permission from J Lonstein. *Moe's Textbook of Scoliosis and Other Spinal Deformities* [3rd ed]. Philadelphia: Saunders, 1995. P 406.)

       c. Tuberculosis
       d. Sacroiliac joint infection
    4. Tumor
       a. Benign bony neoplasm
          (1) Osteoid osteoma
          (2) Osteoblastoma
          (3) Aneurysmal bone cyst
          (4) Eosinophilic granuloma
       b. Malignant bony neoplasm
          (1) Ewing's sarcoma
          (2) Osteogenic sarcoma
          (3) Leukemia
       c. Neural neoplasm
          (1) Glioma
          (2) Epidermoid
          (3) Neuroblastoma
    5. Inflammatory disease
       a. Ankylosing spondylitis
       b. Enteropathic arthritis
    6. Extraspinal origin
       a. Neural
       b. Intestinal
       c. Vascular
       d. Psychological
C. Warning signs of serious underlying disorder
    1. Neurologic abnormality
    2. Repeated interference with function (school, play, sports)
    3. Prolonged stiffness
    4. Fever
    5. Age under 11
D. Workup and treatment. If warning signs are present, aggressive workup, including plain radiographs, bone scan, and MRI, is indicated. If not, close follow-up with appropriate activity modification followed by an exercise program for abdominal and extensor muscles may be used at first. Further tests and treatment should then be undertaken if needed.

Bibliography

Thompson GH. Current concepts review: Back pain in children. *J Bone Joint Surg [Am]* 75:928, 1993.

XIII. Congenital scoliosis
  A. Principles. Congenital scoliosis is a scoliosis due to primary vertebral malformation with unbalanced growth.
    1. Types
       a. Failure of segmentation (bar); most deforming (progression < 5 degrees/year)
       b. Failure of formation (hemivertebra)
          (1) Segmented; normal growth plates on either side (progress < 2 degrees/year)
          (2) Semisegmented
          (3) Unsegmented (nonprogressive)

  2. Progression is greatest in first 2 years of life or in adolescent growth spurt.

B. Associated findings

  1. Spinal dysraphism
  2. VATER syndrome: *V*ertebral anomalies, *A*nal malformations, *C*ardiac defects, *T*racheoesophageal fistula, *R*enal and *R*adial anomalies, and *L*imb malformations
  3. Goldenhar syndrome (oculoauriculovertebral dysplasia)
  4. Arthrogryposis
  5. Multiple pterygium syndrome
  6. Skeletal dysplasia

C. Evaluation

  1. Analyze films from infancy or coned anteroposterior and oblique films
  2. Cardiac auscultation
  3. Renal ultrasound or intravenous pyelogram
  4. MRI if there is neurologic asymmetry, or if surgical instrumentation is planned
  5. Note: Measurement error is greater than in idiopathic scoliosis (i.e., 10–19 degrees)

D. Treatment

  1. Bracing has little or no value.
  2. Document progression with films taken in same position every 6–12 months.
  3. If progressive
    a. Acceptable deformity: fuse in situ (anterior and posterior if well-formed vertebral body)
    b. Unacceptable deformity
      (1) Anteroposterior convex growth arrest if under age 5
      (2) Osteotomy or excision
      (3) Careful instrumentation of flexible segment of curve is an option.

XIV. Scheuermann's kyphosis

A. Definition.
Developmental wedging of three or more adjacent vertebra over 5 degrees constitutes Scheuermann's kyphosis. Incidence is approximately 5% of general population.

B. Clinical features

  1. Thoracic or thoracolumbar kyphosis
  2. Pain within curve, usually during growth spurt
  3. Mild scoliosis may coexist
  4. Tight hamstrings

C. Radiographic findings

  1. Wedging of three or more vertebrae
  2. Irregularity of end plates
  3. Disc space narrowing
  4. Schmorl's nodes

D. Treatment

  1. Exercise program: Strengthen abdominal and hip extensor muscles and stretch hamstrings.
  2. Nonsteroidal anti-inflammatory agents.
  3. Bracing of curve if 50–70 degrees and if skeletal maturity is less than Risser 3.
  4. Operative correction: Optional for curves greater than 65 degrees if pain persists or if deformity is objectionable to patient.

a. Posterior column shortening and fusion alone if flexible.
b. Anterior release and posterior fusion if rigid.

Bibliography

Lowe TG. Current concepts review: Scheuermann's disease. *J Bone Joint Surg [Am]* 72:940, 1990.

XV. Spondylolysis and spondylolisthesis
  A. Principles. Spondylolisthesis is the most common identifiable cause of back pain in children. The prevalence begins to plateau at about 6% by age 6. Etiology is unknown but can be conceptualized as a stress fracture in a susceptible pars interarticularis. The fifth lumbar vertebra is most commonly involved. Twenty percent of cases are unilateral pars defects.
    1. Classification
      a. Dysplastic
      b. Isthmic (most common)
      c. Degenerative
      d. Traumatic
      e. Pathologic
    2. Risk factors for isthmic spondylolysis
      a. Positive family history
      b. Spina bifida occulta of L5
      c. Excessive stress from Scheuermann's kyphosis, gymnastics, athetosis, football lineman activity
    3. Risk factors for progressive slip
      a. Preadolescent age
      b. Female gender
      c. Dysplastic slip
      d. High-grade slip (III or IV)
      e. High slip angle
  B. Signs and symptoms most commonly develop in adolescence.
    1. Symptoms
      a. Low back pain that is activity related and becomes worse with extension
      b. Pain in buttocks or proximal thighs
    2. Signs
      a. Stiff-legged gait or pelvic waddle (absent in many patients)
      b. Limited forward flexion
      c. Prominent ilia, if acute or severe
      d. Palpable step-off of spinous process if slip is greater than 25%
      e. Weakness of ankle or bladder dysfunction (rare)
  C. Plain radiographic findings
    1. Pars defect on lateral film
    2. Pars defect on oblique film (break in "Scottie dog's" neck)
    3. Elongation of pars
    4. Vertebral body slippage (Fig. 2-30 shows measurement technique)

   5. Relative lumbosacral kyphosis (Fig. 2-30)
D. Additional radiographic studies
   1. Bone scan of spine with SPECT if plain films are nega-
       tive or if needed to determine whether condition is
       acute or chronic
   2. CT scan if needed for detail to confirm subtle spondylolysis
   3. MRI if significant neurologic finding exists
E. Treatment
   1. Activity restriction as indicated.
   2. Consider brace treatment for healing of acute slip or if
       symptoms persist.
   3. Strengthen abdominal and extensor muscles.
   4. Fusion if severe pain or symptoms persist or if slip is
       greater than 50%.
   5. Repair (bone graft) of defect if slip is less than 5 mm
       and symptomatic and if patient is under age 25.
   6. Reduction is controversial, usually considered only if slip
       is high grade and deformity is the primary complaint.
   7. Skeletally immature patients should be followed during
       growth to watch for progression.

Bibliography

Hensinger RN. Current concepts review: Spondylolysis and
   spondylolisthesis in children and adolescents. *J Bone Joint
   Surg [Am]* 71:1098, 1989.

XVI. Musculoskeletal tumors
   A. Characteristics. Most pediatric skeletal tumors are
       benign. The most common primary malignancies include
       osteosarcoma, Ewing's sarcoma, and rhabdomyosarcoma.
       Secondary skeletal involvement may occur with leukemia
       and neuroblastoma.
   B. Symptoms. Worrisome symptoms are night pain or pain
       unrelated to activity, rapid increase in pain, increasing
       fatigue, or bruising.
   C. Laboratory studies
       1. Erythrocyte sedimentation rate (ESR) is mildly elevat-
           ed for most malignant tumors.
       2. CBC is abnormal in leukemia and lymphoma.
   D. Radiologic studies
       1. Plain films: Location, morphology, and host reaction are
           the most diagnostic features.
       2. Radionuclide scans are very sensitive for malignant
           bone and soft tissue tumors but may be negative in
           eosinophilic granuloma.
       3. CT scan is best when bony changes need to be better
           defined.
       4. MRI shows bony detail less well but soft-tissue and
           intramedullary detail well.
   E. Tumor types (Fig. 2-31)
       1. Benign
           a. Eosinophilic granuloma: reticuloendothelial lesion
               usually centrally located in one or several bones;

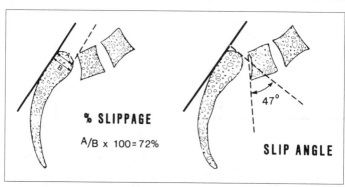

Fig. 2-30. *(Left)* Vertebral body slippage. Measurement of percent slip is performed with respect to a line drawn from the posterior cortex of the sacrum proximally. Note that the reference line from the superior vertebra is parallel to the sacral line, not to the L5 cortex. (A = distance from posterior cortex of sacrum to posterior-inferior corner of L5; B = width of S1.) *(Right)* Measurement of slip angle (lumbosacral kyphosis). Note that the sacral reference line is drawn perpendicular to the posterior cortex because the sacral end plate may be rounded. (Reproduced with permission from J Lonstein. *Moe's Textbook of Scoliosis and Other Spinal Deformities* [3rd ed]. Philadelphia: Saunders, 1995. P 406.)

    poorly or well circumscribed. Usually waxes and wanes spontaneously.

b. Osteoid osteoma: Painful nidus surrounded by sclerosis. Ages 6–25.

c. Osteochondroma (osteocartilaginous exostosis): metaphyseal, solitary, or multiple; ceases growth at maturity.

d. Chondromyxoid fibroma: eccentric local lesion, usually in lower extremity; progressively enlarging. Ages 10–25.

e. Chondroblastoma: epiphyseal tumor of adolescence; lucent with foci of internal calcification.

f. Unicameral bone cyst (UBC): central lucent metaphyseal lesion usually of proximal humerus or femur; expands and thins cortex; resolves at maturity.

g. Nonossifying fibroma (NOF): eccentric intracortical defect in metaphysis; resolves by maturity.

h. Adamantinoma: sclerotic anterior cortical defect, usually of tibia.

i. Enchondroma: central lucent defect with internal calcification.

j. Giant-cell tumor: lucent epimetaphyseal tumor appears just after maturity.

k. Aneurysmal bone cyst: expansile metaphyseal lesion of late adolescence destroys cortex but leaves thin shell.

2. Malignant

    a. Fibrosarcoma

    b. Osteosarcoma: the most common primary malignant bone tumor; metaphyseal; located in fastest-growing regions.

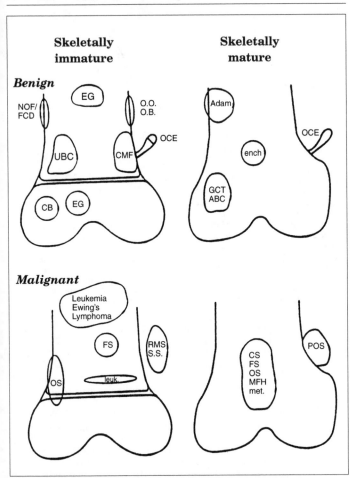

Fig. 2-31. Sites of musculoskeletal tumors in skeletally immature and skeletally mature children. Benign: EG = eosinophilic granuloma; OO/OB = osteoid osteoma or osteoblastoma; OCE = osteocartilaginous exostasis; CMF = chondromyxofibroma; CB = chondroblastoma; UBC = unicameral bone cyst, NOF/FCD = nonossifying fibroma or fibrous cortical defect; Adam = adamantinoma; Ench = enchondroma; GCT = giant-cell tumor; ABC = aneurysmal bone cyst. Malignant: FS = fibrosarcoma; OS = osteosarcoma, CS = chondrosarcoma, MFH = malignant fibrous histiocytoma, POS = parosteal osteosarcoma, Meta = metastasis, SS = synovial sarcoma, RMS = rhabdomyosarcoma.

    c. Chondrosarcoma: central or peripheral expansile tumor of young adults.

    d. Ewing's sarcoma: small-cell tumor of diaphysis; ages 5–15; usually lytic with extensive periosteal reaction.

F. Tumors common to specific locations in children

  1. Long bones (see Fig. 2-31)

  2. Spine

    a. Posterior elements

      (1) Aneurysmal bone cyst

      (2) Osteoid osteoma

      (3) Osteoblastoma

    b. Anterior elements

      (1) Histiocytosis

      (2) Hemangioma

      (3) Osteosarcoma

      (4) Ewing's sarcoma

      (5) Chordoma

  3. Ribs

    a. Fibrous dysplasia

    b. Ewing's sarcoma

    c. Chondrosarcoma

    d. Metastasis

  4. Pelvis

    a. Ewing's sarcoma

    b. Fibrous dysplasia

    c. Aneurysmal bone cyst

    d. Osteoblastoma

    e. Eosinophilic granuloma

    f. Leukemia

    g. Osteosarcoma

  5. Scapula

    a. Ewing's sarcoma

    b. Osteoblastoma

    c. Aneurysmal bone cyst

G. Staging

  1. Malignant tumors (Table 2-3)

  2. Benign tumors

    a. Latent

    b. Active

    c. Aggressive; may expand into soft tissues or metastasize

Table 2-3. Malignant tumors

Surgical stage	Surgical grade (G)	Site (T)	Metastases (M)	
I_A	Low (G_1)	Intracompartmental (T_1)	M0	B
	Low (G_1)	Extracompartmental (T_2)	M0	
II_A	High (G_2)	Intracompartmental (T_1)	M0	
	High (G_2)	Extracompartmental (T_2)	M0	
III	Any	Any T	M_1	

Source: WJ Enneking. *Musculoskeletal Tumor Surgery*. New York: Churchill Livingstone, 1983.

XVII. Musculoskeletal problems in hemophilia

A. Characteristics. Hemophilia A (factor VIII deficiency) and B (factor IX deficiency) are the two most common bleeding disorders, followed by von Willebrand's disease. A factor level below 5% of normal risks serious bleeding. These conditions should be jointly managed by hematologists and orthopedic specialists.

B. Factor doses and kinetics

Factor	Percent rise after l unit/kg dose	Half-life (approximately)
VIII	2	12 h
IX	1	24 h

C. Treatment of acute hemarthropathy
  1. Factor replacement 50% q48h × 6 days.
  2. Aspirate.
  3. Immobilize.
  4. Rehabilitate according to symptoms.

D. Treatment of subacute hemarthropathy
  1. Factor replacement 30% × 2–6 weeks.
  2. Strengthen and increase range of motion.

E. Control of bleeding after fracture
  1. Factor replacement 50% × 1–2 days, then:
  2. Factor replacement 30% × 1 week.

F. Radiographic evaluation
  1. The **Arnold classification** is the most conceptually logical.

I	Soft-tissue swelling
II	Osteopenia, epiphyseal overgrowth
III	Subchondral cysts, wide/square contours
IV	Joint space narrow, irregular
V	Joint space absent

  2. The **Greene classification,** a 4-part, 7-point scheme, is more reproducible for research purposes but less meaningful for individual patient.

Greene classification	Points
Subchondral irregularity	
Absent	0
Mild (< 50% of the joint surface)	1
Pronounced	2
Narrowing of the joint space	
Absent	0
< 50%	1
> 50%	2
Erosion of the joint margin	
Absent	0
Present	1
Incongruity of the joint surfaces	
Absent	0
Mild	1
Pronounced	2

G. Control of subacute hemarthropathy
  1. Chronic factor replacement

2. Splinting
3. Cast
4. Synovectomy; arthroscopy or radionuclide dose

Bibliography

Greene WB, Yankuskar BC, Guilford WB et al. Comparison of radiological classification of hemophilia with clinical parameters. *J Bone Joint Surg [Am]* 71:237, 1989.

XVIII. Infections of bone and joint
    A. Evaluation and workup. Obtain all necessary cultures before starting antibiotics.
        1. Blood cultures in all patients if possible
        2. Spinal tap if indicated
        3. Aspirate bone or joint
        4. Bone scan if location difficult on physical examination
    B. Differential diagnosis
        1. Transient synovitis
        2. Postinfectious arthritis
        3. Juvenile rheumatoid arthritis
        4. Ewing's sarcoma
        5. Rheumatic fever
    C. Treatment. Antibiotic recommendations by age (Table 2-4).
    D. Organism. The type of organism causing bone and joint infection in children varies with age, but staph is the most common organism at all ages. Figures 2-32, 2-33, and 2-34 give specifics by age.

Table 2-4. Antibiotic recommendations by age

Age	Septic arthritis	Osteomyelitis
<1 mo	Oxacillin and gentamicin or cefotaxime	Oxacillin and gentamicin or cefotaxime
1 mo–4 yrs	Cefuroxime	Oxacillin, first-generation cephalosporin, or clindamycin
>4 yrs	Oxacillin, first-generation cephalosporin, or clindamycin	Oxacillin, first-generation cephalosporin, or clindamycin

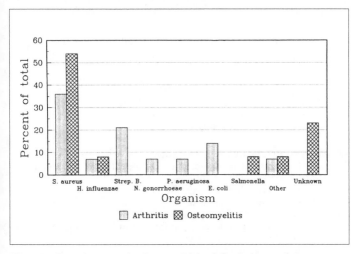

Fig. 2-32. Organisms causing bone and joint infection in newborns. Osteomyelitis and septic arthritis portrayed separately. (Data from MA Jackson, JD Nelson. Etiology and management of acute suppurative bone and joint infections in pediatric patients. *J Pediatr Orthop* **2:313, 1982.)**

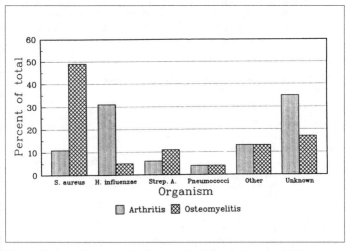

Fig. 2-33. Organisms causing bone and joint infection in children age 1 month to 5 years. (Data from MA Jackson, JD Nelson. Etiology and management of acute suppurative bone and joint infections in pediatric patients. *J Pediatr Orthop* **2:313, 1982.)**

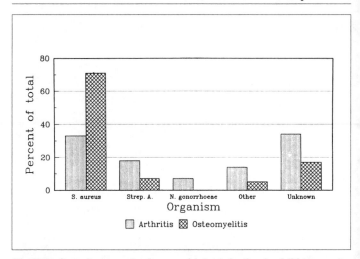

Fig. 2-34. Organisms causing bone and joint infection in children age 5 and up. (Data from MA Jackson, JD Nelson. Etiology and management of acute suppurative bone and joint infections in pediatric patients. *J Pediatr Orthop* 2:313, 1982.)

Skeletal Syndromes and Systemic Disorders in Children's Orthopedics

Developmental syndromes involving skeletal abnormalities are often encountered unexpectedly. A diagnosis or discussion of prognosis may be called for when the physician has no opportunity to consult definitive references. Diagnosis requires knowledge of a large number of facts rather than basic principles, and this chapter can help the physician in these cases. The information is organized according to presenting features. For a more detailed discussion of any of these conditions, consult one of the references listed at the end of the chapter.

Chapter Outline

I. Skeletal dysplasias. Skeletal dysplasias involve basic and systemic abnormalities of bone and cartilage growth and development, usually causing short stature.

A. Diagnosis of skeletal dysplasias

  1. Height and proportion

    a. Birth length

    b. Current height and percentile

      (1) Most skeletal dysplasias produce adult height under 60 inches.

      (2) Mean adult height in achondroplasia for males is 52 in. (+ 2 SD = 56 in.) and for females is 50 in. (+ 2 SD = 52 in.).

      (3) Mean adult height in diastrophic dwarfism is 42 in.

    c. Body proportion is determined by comparing limb and trunk lengths.

      (1) Limb height $\approx$ lower segment = symphysis to soles of feet.

      (2) Trunk height $\approx$ upper segment = total height minus lower segment.

      (3) For a graph of normal values by age, see the *Harriet Lane Handbook*.

      (4) Another approach to determining body proportion is to subtract total height from arm span (fingertip to fingertip). Values for normal stature by this measure are –2 cm (–$^{13}/_{16}$ in.) (before age 8), + 1 cm (+ ⅜ in.) (adult females), and + 5 cm (+ 2 in.) (adult males).

    d. Limb segment ratios are best calculated from x-rays.

      (1) Normal ratio of radius to humerus is 75%.

      (2) Normal ratio of tibia to femur is 82%.

      (3) Types of disproportion include rhizomelic (short humerus and femur), mesomelic (short forearms and legs), and acromelic (short hands and feet).

  2. Dysmorphism is morphologic variation of bone and soft tissue that may characterize a specific disorder.

    a. Depressed nasal bridge often seen in achondroplasia.

    b. Long philtrum suggests trichorhinophalangeal dysplasia.

    c. Short broad thumb suggests multiple epiphyseal dysplasia.

    d. V-shaped phalanges suggests trichorhinophalangeal dysplasia.

    e. "Hitchhiker's" thumb and abducted great toe indicates diastrophic dysplasia.

  3. Radiographic evaluation should include these five key studies.

    a. Lateral skull and cervical spine

    b. Lateral lumbar spine

    c. Anteroposterior pelvis

    d. Anteroposterior knees

    e. Anteroposterior hand and wrist

  4. Family evaluation

    a. Construct pedigree of at least all first-degree relatives.

    b. If family history is negative, consider the following:

      (1) New mutation

      (2) Gonadal mutation

        (3) Recessive trait

        (4) Nonpaternity

   5. Laboratory evaluation is usually not indicated but can be useful if prior workup is negative. It should include the following studies:

     a. Chemistry profile

     b. Endocrine evaluation

     c. Urine workup for storage disorder

B. Achondroplasia

     a. Achondroplasia is autosomal dominant but usually due to frequent new mutation. It is the most common skeletal dysplasia.

     b. Major features

        (1) Midface hypoplasia

        (2) Rhizomelic dwarfism

        (3) Genu varum (variable)

        (4) Three- to 6-month delay in motor milestones

        (5) Thoracolumbar kyphosis, often resolving with growth

        (6) Spinal stenosis. This is greatest in lumbar spine and distally but may affect entire spine, including foramen magnum, and cause severe developmental delay.

     c. Height (Fig. 3-1). Final height for males is 46–56 in., and for females, 44–55 in.

C. Pseudoachondroplasia

   1. Although these patients are also rhizomelic, the epiphyseal involvement in this syndrome causes basic differences from achondroplasia.

   2. Major features

     a. Rhizomelic shortening of extremities

     b. Variable knee deformities (varus on one side, valgus on the other)

     c. Mild platyspondyly, minimal scoliosis, no stenosis

     d. Odontoid hypoplasia, C1–C2 instability

     e. Epiphyseal deformation; eventual degeneration

     f. Ligamentous laxity

D. Diastrophic dysplasia

   1. Autosomal recessive

   2. Major features

     a. "Cauliflower ear" develops at approximately 6 months

     b. Rhizomelic shortening of extremities

     c. Contractures of major joints with later degenerative joint disease (DJD)

     d. Hands: hitchhiker's thumb, symphalangism

     e. Dislocated hips (occasionally)

     f. Equinovarus foot deformities

     g. Cervical spina bifida with kyphosis; sometimes resolves

     h. Scoliosis of thoracic and lumbar spine

E. Spondyloepiphyseal dysplasia congenita

   1. Autosomal dominant with frequent new mutations

   2. Major features

     a. Odontoid hypoplasia or os odontoideum; may have instability

     b. Platyspondyly, scoliosis

     c. Coxa vara, epiphyseal irregularity, DJD

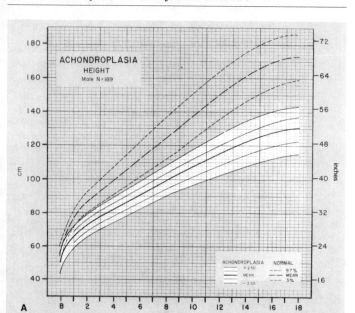

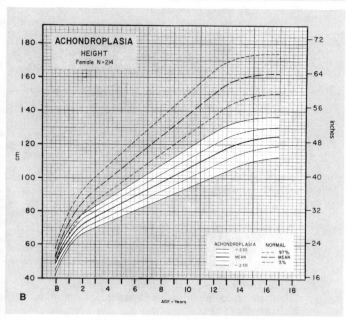

Fig. 3-1. Comparison of growth patterns of normal and achondroplasic persons. A. Males. B. Females. (Reproduced with permission from WA Horton. Growth in achondroplasia. *J Pediatr* **93**:436, 1978.)

F. Spondyloepiphyseal dysplasia tarda

1. Variable transmission; diagnosis late in childhood
2. Major features
   a. Irregular ossification, DJD
   b. Hips may resemble Perthes disease but are bilaterally synchronous.
   c. Scoliosis
   d. Occasional cervical instability

G. Multiple epiphyseal dysplasia

1. Autosomal dominant
2. Major features
   a. Variable, usually mild short stature due to short limbs
   b. Irregular epiphyseal ossification with deformity, pain, DJD
   c. Hips, knees, and ankles are most involved.
   d. Usually presents in late childhood to adulthood

H. Metatropic dysplasia. Major features:

1. Epiphyseal or metaphyseal enlargement: "knobby" joints with contractures
2. Cervical stenosis, instability
3. Scoliosis, kyphosis, later onset
4. Coccygeal tail
5. Thoracic hypoplasia; may cause respiratory compromise
6. Initially short-limb dwarfism; becomes short-trunk type with onset of scoliosis

I. Chondrodysplasia punctata (Conradi-Hünermann syndrome)

1. Autosomal dominant
2. **Major features**
   a. Multiple asymmetric epiphyseal calcifications
   b. Good prognosis

J. Multiple osteocartilaginous exostoses

1. Autosomal dominant
2. Clinical appearance features mild short stature. Categories of problems:
   a. Local impingement on tendons, nerves, spinal canal, and ribs
   b. Asymmetric growth in two-bone segments leading to valgus knees, ankles, elbows, and wrists and possibly to radial head dislocation
   c. Leg length inequality (usually < 4 cm)
   d. Risk of malignant degeneration (about 1% of patients)
3. **Radiographic features**
   a. Osteochondromas in metaphysis, pointing away from joint
   b. Cortex of osteochondroma is confluent with that of host bone
   c. May be sessile or pedunculated
4. **Treatment**
   a. Resect lesions only when symptomatic. Resection does not predictably increase forearm rotation.
   b. Correct knee and ankle valgus when greater than 10 degrees.
   c. Monitor in adulthood every 2 years with bone scan.

K. Dysplasia epiphysealis hemimelica (Trevor's disease)
   1. Definition: epiphyseal osteochondroma; no genetic pattern
   2. Clinical features
      a. Presents in first decade
      b. Restricted joint motion
      c. Enlarged joint or locked joint
      d. Knee, foot, and ankle are most commonly involved
   3. Radiographic features include multiple opacities in exostotic cartilage; these eventually coalesce.
   4. Treatment: resection, attempting to preserve normal cartilage.
L. Multiple enchondromas (Ollier's disease)
   1. Clinical presentation
      a. Angular deformity
      b. Bony irregularity
      c. Limb length inequality
   2. Radiographic features
      a. Diffuse enchondromas in metaphysis; occasionally epiphyses. Usually asymmetric.
      b. Treatment
         (1) Angular or length correction of limb
         (2) Monitor for malignancy, especially in Maffucci's syndrome
M. Cleidocranial dysplasia
      a. Autosomal dominant
      b. Persistently open skull sutures with bulging calvarium
      c. Hypoplasia or aplasia of clavicles
      d. Wide symphysis pubis
      e. Hip abnormalities
      f. Short middle phalanx of fifth finger
      g. Syringomyelia may be present.
N. Dyschondrosteosis. Major features:
   1. Madelung's deformity
   2. Relative shortening of forearm and leg
   3. Females predominate

Bibliography

Green MG. *Harriet Lane Handbook*. Chicago: Year Book, 1991.

Jensen BL. Somatic development in cleidocranial dysplasia. *Am J Med Genet* 35:69, 1990.

Kettelkamp DB, Campbell CJ, Bonfiglio M et al. Dysplasia epiphysealis hemimelica. *J Bone Joint Surg [Am]* 48:746, 1966.

II. Other syndromes involving short stature
A. Cornelia de Lange syndrome
   1. Major features
      a. Synophrys (single confluent eyebrow)
      b. Down-turned mouth
      c. Mandibular spur, in infancy
      d. Hirsutism
      e. Gastroesophageal reflux

      f. Small for gestational age, with continued growth retardation

      g. Motor and intellectual delay

      h. Cardiac abnormalities

  2. Orthopedic involvement

      a. Upper-extremity anomalies in almost all patients

      b. Micromelia, phocomelia

      c. Decreased number of fingers

      d. Lobster claw hand

      e. Proximally placed thumb

      f. Elbow anomalies

  3. Lower extremities

      a. Miscellaneous foot deformities and contracture

      b. Avascular necrosis of femoral head in 10%

  4. Treatment: Correct lower-extremity abnormalities if limiting ambulation. Individualized treatment for upper extremities.

B. Riley-Day familial dysautonomia

  1. Ashkenazi Jews only; autosomal recessive

  2. Sympathetic overactivity is key feature.

  3. Major features

      a. Deficient sensation of pain and proprioception

      b. Gastroesophageal reflux, pneumonia

      c. Variable life expectancy

  4. Orthopedic abnormalities and implications

      a. Scoliosis or kyphosis before age 8; poor brace tolerance; fuse early

      b. Fractures due to osteopenia or dyscoordination

      c. Avascular necrosis of femoral head, distal femur, talus

      d. Hip dysplasia

C. Nail-patella syndrome

  1. Autosomal dominant, normal life expectancy.

  2. Orthopedic features

      a. Nails grooved, small, or absent, especially on thumb

      b. Multiple knee anomalies: patella tripartite, small, or absent; lateral femoral condyle hypoplastic; osteochondritis dissecans of lateral femur and talus

  3. Elbow: capitellar hypoplasia, cubitus valgus, flexion contracture

  4. Iliac horns

III. Sclerosing bone disorders

A. Fibrodysplasia ossificans progressiva

  1. Progressive, disabling heterotopic ossification or ankylosis

  2. Characteristic shortening or valgus of great toe

  3. Ossification starts as tender, hard nodule; progresses proximal to distal, posterior to anterior

  4. Do not biopsy—this may accelerate the process.

  5. Genetics: usually a spontaneous mutation, but it may be transmitted as autosomal dominant

B. Progressive diaphyseal dysplasia

  1. Clinical features: pain, fatigue, muscle atrophy

  2. Radiographic features: symmetrically widened, sclerotic diaphyses; epiphyses spared; tibia and femur most commonly involved.

  3. Treatment: osteotomies only if there is marked deformity

C. **Melorheostosis**

1. A syndrome involving asymmetric, extraosseous, longitudinal hyperostotic streaks; limb pain and soft-tissue contracture.

2. Treatment: analgesics, bracing, contracture releases, and bone shortening

D. **Osteopathia striata**

1. Linear intraosseous metaphyseal striations

2. Autosomal dominant

3. Asymptomatic

4. No treatment required

E. **Osteopoikilosis**

1. Multiple symmetric intraosseous epiphyseal or metaphyseal "spots"

2. Autosomal dominant

3. Asymptomatic

IV. **Marfanoid disorders**

A. **Marfan syndrome.** This disorder of fibrillin has multiple effects on the skeleton and connective tissue. Because some features may be seen in the general population, the following diagnostic criteria have been developed.

1. **Diagnostic criteria.** Positive family history or skeletal involvement.

2. Involvement of two other systems—at least one must be a major manifestation (see * below).

3. System involvement (* indicates major manifestation).

   a. Skeletal

       (1) Anterior chest deformity

       (2) Dolichostenomelia (long, narrow limbs)

       (3) Arachnodactyly (long, narrow digits)

       (4) Vertebral column deformity (kyphosis, scoliosis)

       (5) Tall stature

       (6) High, narrowly arched palate

       (7) Increased appendicular joint mobility

       (8) Protrusio acetabuli

   b. Ocular

       (1) *Ectopia lentis (superolateral lens dislocation)

       (2) Flat cornea

       (3) Retinal detachment

       (4) Myopia

   c. Cardiovascular

       (1) *Ascending aortic aneurysm with dilation of valsalva sinuses

       (2) *Aortic dissection, usually ascending segment

       (3) Aortic valve regurgitation

       (4) Mitral valve regurgitation

       (5) Abdominal aortic aneurysm

   d. Pulmonary

       (1) Spontaneous pneumothorax

       (2) Apical bleb

   e. Skin

       (1) Striae atrophicae (stretch marks)

       (2) Hernia

   f. Central nervous system

       (1) *Dural ectasia

(2) Learning disability

(3) Hyperactivity

4. Implications

a. Monitor aortic and cardiac status

b. Beta blocker for aortic dilation

c. Restrict from vigorous exertion

d. Counsel regarding genetics

e. Treat skeletal deformity if symptomatic

B. Homocystinuria

1. Homocystinuria may be mistaken for Marfan syndrome, but it is most readily distinguished by mental retardation. It has the following major features:

a. Mental retardation

b. Dislocated lens (inferomedial)

c. Arachnodactyly

d. Joint stiffness

e. Cavus feet

f. Scoliosis or kyphosis

2. Diagnosis: urine amino acid screen

3. Treatment: vitamin B_6 administration, methionine restriction

C. Congenital contractural arachnodactyly. This is also a Marfan look-alike; so much so that Marfan's original patient had this syndrome. Clinical features:

1. Face: oval with recessed jaw, flattened ear

2. Eyes: occasional intraocular coloboma

3. Heart: congenital septal and valve defects

4. Skeleton

a. Flexion contracture that partially improves with time

b. Hands: contracture of proximal interphalangeal (PIP) and distal interphalangeal (DIP) joints

c. Scoliosis: appears by mid-childhood

D. Achard syndrome. Clinical features:

1. Arachnodactyly

2. Generalized ligamentous laxity

3. Mandibular hypoplasia

E. Stickler syndrome (hereditary arthro-ophthalmopathy)

1. **Etiology.** A mutation in type II collagen. Abraham Lincoln may have had hereditary arthro-ophthalmopathy.

2. **Clinical features**

a. Progressive myopia beginning in first decade

b. Retinal detachment

c. Abnormal epiphyseal development, eventual DJD

d. Mild joint hypermobility in some cases

e. Marfanoid habitus in some cases

f. Autosomal dominant

Bibliography

Beals RK. Hereditary arthro-ophthalmopathy. *Clin Orthop* 125:32, 1977.

V. Arthrogryposis or contracture

A. Arthrogryposis multiplex congenita. This is the classic contractural syndrome seen by orthopedists. The etiology is unknown; it is probably multifactorial. Major features are all skeletal: It may affect all four limbs, upper extremities only, or lower extremities only. Involvement is usually greatest distally within each limb.

1. Hips are frequently dislocated. Contractures are usually into abduction and external rotation
2. Knees: flexion more common than extension
3. Clubfoot and vertical talus are common, often resistant to cast treatment
4. Upper extremities: extended at elbows, adducted, stiff fingers
5. Spine: paralytic scoliosis, torticollis
6. Implications for treatment
   a. Range of motion can be shifted but not increased
   b. Osteotomies most useful near end of growth
   c. Fractures common after manipulation or cast

B. Larsen syndrome

1. Orthopedic features
   a. Dislocated hips, hyperextended or dislocated knees
   b. Clubfeet
   c. Normal muscle mass
   d. Elbow dislocations
   e. Cervical kyphosis and instability
   f. Thoracic and lumbar scoliosis
2. Nonorthopedic features
   a. Flattened face, depressed nasal bridge
   b. Cleft palate

C. Freeman-Sheldon (whistling face) syndrome

1. Small mouth and chin (may cause difficulty with intubation)
2. Arthrogrypotic, flexed, and ulnar-deviated fingers
3. Clubfeet or vertical talus
4. Scoliosis or kyphosis

D. Möbius syndrome

1. Congenital facial diplegia
2. Variable absence of shoulder girdle muscles
3. Clubfeet and hand contractures or anomalies

E. Pterygium syndromes

1. Multiple pterygium syndrome
   a. Static disorder with flexion contractures and webs at all flexion creases
   b. Short stature
   c. Congenital spinal anomalies
2. Popliteal pterygium syndrome
   a. Webs only across perineum and knees
   b. Facial malformations
   c. Contractures are due to a single cord from ischium to calcaneus, with the nerve bow-strung across the joint

VI. Vascular abnormalities

A. Klippel-Trenaunay-Weber syndrome

1. Clinical features
   a. Cutaneous hemangioma (port-wine stain)
   b. Varicose veins

        c. Limb hemi-hypertrophy: often nonlinear growth pattern

   2. Treatment

      a. Initially treated with compressive therapy

      b. May have specific indications for surgery

B. Maffucci syndrome. Major features:

   1. Multiple enchondromas

   2. Cavernous hemangiomas

   3. Risk of sarcomatous transformation

C. Sturge-Weber syndrome. Major features:

   1. Port-wine hemangioma in trigeminal distribution

   2. Neurologic sequelae due to meningeal hemangioma

D. Blue-rubber bleb nevus syndrome

   1. Autosomal dominant

   2. Clinical features

      a. Bluish cavernous hemangiomas on trunk and upper arms; may bleed from GI tract locations; may cause pain.

      b. Regional hyperhidrosis

E. Kasabach-Merritt syndrome. Clinical features:

   1. Solitary or multiple cavernous hemangiomas on trunk or extremities

   2. Consumptive coagulopathy secondary to hemangiomas

F. Ataxia-telangiectasia (Louis-Bar syndrome). Clinical features:

   1. Telangiectasia on conjunctivae, face, neck, and arms

   2. Progressive ataxia

   3. Genetics: autosomal dominant

VII. Overgrowth syndromes

A. Generalized bodily overgrowth

   1. Prader-Willi syndrome

      a. Partial deletion of chromosome 15

      b. Major findings

         (1) Infantile hypotonia

         (2) Obesity beginning after age 1

         (3) Mental retardation

         (4) Cryptorchidism

         (5) Short stature

         (6) Eyes slant upward and lateral

      c. Orthopedic findings

         (1) Developmental dysplasia of the hip in 10%

         (2) Scoliosis in 50%

         (3) Small hands and feet

   2. Bardet-Biedl syndrome

      a. Etiology unknown; genetics probably autosomal recessive

      b. Major findings

         (1) Truncal obesity

         (2) Mental retardation

         (3) Hypogonadism

         (4) Retinitis pigmentosa

         (5) Renal abnormalities

      c. Orthopedic abnormalities: postaxial polydactyly (feet more than hands)

   3. Beckwith-Wiedemann syndrome

      a. Autosomal dominant

      b. Major findings
- **(1)** Large stature
- **(2)** Omphalocele
- **(3)** Macroglossia (may partially regress)
- **(4)** Hypoglycemia
- **(5)** Multiple organ enlargement; risk of Wilms' tumor

      c. Orthopedic abnormalities
- **(1)** Leg length inequality
- **(2)** Neurologic damage if hypoglycemia not controlled
- **(3)** Polydactyly, idiopathic scoliosis, radial head dislocation variable

B. Asymmetric overgrowth

1. Idiopathic hemihypertrophy

      a. Skeletal findings
- **(1)** One side of body larger in all dimensions
- **(2)** Growth proportionate over time
- **(3)** Lower extremities most often affected; trunk and upper extremities may be affected

      b. Genitourinary system
- **(1)** Wilms' tumor (nephroblastoma) in approximately 5%
- **(2)** Medullary sponge kidney
- **(3)** Renal malposition

      c. Vascular system: aortic, cerebral vascular, or congenital heart abnormalities

2. Russell-Silver syndrome

      a. Short stature

      b. Small, triangular face; may be asymmetric

      c. Genitourinary system and genital malformations

      d. Orthopedic features
- **(1)** Hemihypertrophy
- **(2)** Other miscellaneous skeletal findings

3. Goldenhar syndrome

      a. Major features
- **(1)** Epibulbar dermoids
- **(2)** Preauricular skin tags, facial asymmetry

      b. Orthopedic abnormalities
- **(1)** Congenital vertebral anomalies
- **(2)** Other aspects of VATER syndrome association

      c. Implications: Monitor for scoliosis; be aware of difficult intubation.

4. Klippel-Feil syndrome

      a. Key feature: cervical spine fusions; may have stenosis, instability

      b. Possible skeletal associations
- **(1)** Congenital or "idiopathic" scoliosis of lower spine (60% of patients)
- **(2)** Sprengel's deformity (30% of patients)
- **(3)** Upper extremity or hand anomalies

      c. Nonskeletal associations
- **(1)** Genitourinary or renal malformations
- **(2)** Hearing impairment
- **(3)** Cardiac anomalies
- **(4)** Facial asymmetry

      d. Implications

(1) Screen early for hearing impairment, genitourinary malformations (ultrasound)
(2) Counsel regarding activity and anesthesia if neck is unstable

5. Proteus syndrome
    a. A hemartomatous disorder affecting all three germ layers.
    b. Characterized by its variability; named for the Greek god able to change shape at will.
    c. Macrodactyly and asymmetric tissue overgrowth are key features.
    d. Diagnosis can be established by adding up the points assigned to each criterion below for a total score:

Diagnostic criteria	Points
Macrodactyly, hemihypertrophy, or both	5
Thickening of skin	4
Lipomas and subcutaneous tumors	4
Verrucous epidermal nevus	3
Macrocephaly, irregular skull	2.5
Other minor abnormalities	1

Definitive diagnosis is made if score is 13 points or higher; questionable diagnosis is 10–13 points; diagnosis excluded is less than 10 points.

VIII. Neurofibromatosis

  A. Neurofibromatosis is the most prevalent skeletal disorder to be caused by a single gene defect. It is a hemartomatous disorder, probably of neural crest origin.
  B. Diagnosis is established when the patient meets at least two of the following NIH criteria.
    1. Café au lait spots (5 or more spots >1.5 cm after puberty or > 0.5 cm before puberty)
    2. Subcutaneous neurofibroma
    3. Positive biopsy
    4. Positive family history (first-degree relative affected)
    5. Skeletal manifestations
      a. Long bone pseudarthrosis
      b. Dystrophic curve of spine
      c. Elephantiasis neuromatosa
    6. Optic glioma
    7. Two or more Lisch nodules (hamartomas in iris)
    8. Axillary or inguinal freckling
  C. Features of dystrophic spinal curve
    1. Severe apical rotation or wedging
    2. Paravertebral mass
    3. "Spindling" of transverse process
    4. Thinning of rib
    5. Enlargement of the foramen
    6. Vertebral scalloping
  D. Orthopedic implications
    1. Dystrophic curves require more aggressive treatment than nondystrophic curves. (Fuse if >30 degrees; anterior and posterior fusion if >70 degrees or if kyphosis >50 degrees. Explore fusion postoperatively.)
    2. Preoperative CT scan or myelogram on all dystrophic curves.

      3. Rule out sarcoma if unexplained pain or localized growth occurs.

IX. Ehlers-Danlos syndromes. This group of connective tissue abnormalities includes at least 11 different subtypes. Many other patients do not fit precisely into one of the groups. The Ehlers-Danlos syndromes are best illustrated in table form (Table 3-1).

X. Osteogenesis imperfecta

  A. A group of disorders of type II collagen causing bone fragility and in some cases blue sclerae, hearing loss, and abnormal dentin. The osseous fragility tends to improve after puberty.

  B. Sillence types

    1. Type I

      a. Variable osseous fragility (minimal through moderately severe)

      b. Distinctly blue sclerae (at all ages)

      c. Presenile hearing loss

      d. Autosomal dominant

    2. Type II (lethal perinatal osteogenesis imperfecta)

      a. Extremely severe osseous fragility, with stillbirth or neonatal death.

      b. Subgroup A: Radiographs show broad, crumpled long bones and broad ribs with continuous beading. Autosomal dominant or new mutation.

      c. Subgroup B: Radiographs show broad, crumpled long bones; ribs show discontinuous beading or are not beaded. Autosomal recessive.

      d. Subgroup C: Radiographs show thin, fractured long bones and thin, beaded ribs. Autosomal recessive (?).

    3. Type III

      a. Autosomal recessive

      b. Fractures at birth, then progressive deformity

      c. Normal sclerae and hearing

    4. Type IV

      a. Moderate osseous fragility

      b. Normal sclerae (blue in infancy)

      c. Variable deformity of long bones and spine

      d. Autosomal dominant

      Note: The value of opalescent dentin for subcategorization of osteogenesis imperfecta is uncertain.

Bibliography

Sillence DO. Osteogenesis imperfecta: An expanding panorama of variants. *Clin Orthop* 159:11, 1981.

XI. Mucopolysaccharidoses. These disorders of mucopolysaccharide storage are all autosomal recessive. They have delayed appearance of signs and symptoms, and most are progressive. Table 3-2 describes their features.

XII. Malformations of the hand and foot

  A. Syndactyly

Table 3-1. Connective tissue abnormalities

Names	Type	Genetics	Skeletal manifestations			Other problems
			Dislocations	Joint laxity	Scoliosis	
Gravis	1	AD	+	+	+	Aneurysms, viscus rupture, hernias
Mitis	2	AD	−	±	−	—
Benign hypermobile	3	AD	+	+	−	Mitral prolapse
Ecchymotic	4	AD/AR	+	Fingers	−	Aneurysms, spontaneous rupture
X-linked	5	X	−	−	−	Intramuscular hemorrhage, "floppy baby"
Ocular-scoliotic	6	AR	+	+	++	Ocular complications
Arthrochalasis multiplex	7	AR	+	+	+	Short stature
Periodontosis	8	AD	−	±	−	Necrobiosis of skin, periodontosis
Occipital horns	9	X	+	+	−	Occipital horns, skeletal dysplasia
Platelet dysfunction	10	AR	−	−	−	Platelet defect
Familial joint laxity	11	AD	Patellae, hips	+	−	—

+ = present feature; ++ = marked feature; − = absent feature; ± = variable; AD = autosomal dominant; AR = autosomal recessive; X = linked to X chromosome.

Table 3-2. Features of muscopolysaccharidoses

Number	Name	Genetics	Enzyme defect	Clinical features
I-H	Hurler	AR	α-L-iduronidase	Diagnosis at 1–3 yrs of age, corneal clouding, mental retardation, kyphoscoliosis
I-S	Scheie	AR	α-L-iduronidase	Corneal clouding, aortic abnormality, normal intelligence, longer survival
II	Hunter	XR	Iduronate sulfate sulfatase	Clear cornea, mild mental retardation, ± kyphosis
III	San fillipo A, B, C, D	AR	—	Dementia, seizures
IV-A	Morquio A	AR	β-galactosidase-6-sulfate sulfatase (increased urinary keratan sulfate)	Short trunk, odontoid hypoplasia with cervical instability, flame-shaped vertebra, kyphosis (thoracolumbar)
IV-B	Morquio B	AR	β-galactosidase	Milder form of IV-A
VI	Maroteaux-Lamy	AR	Arylsulfatase B	Corneal clouding, normal intelligence, ± cervical stenosis, ± thorocolumbar kyphosis
VII	Sly	AR	β-glucuronidase	May have epiphyseal dysplasia

AR = autosomal recessive; XR = X-linked recessive.

1. Terminology
   a. Extent: partial or complete
   b. Simple: skin only
   c. Complex: synostosis
   d. Polysyndactyly: hidden duplicated skeletal structures
2. Isolated syndactyly
   a. Of the five types, long-ring syndactyly is the most common
   b. Look for duplicated phalanges, abnormalities of metacarpals or metatarsals
   c. Autosomal dominant
   d. Minimal risk of associated anomalies
3. Poland syndrome
   a. Simple syndactyly of variable number of fingers
   b. Short fingers (absent or hypoplastic middle phalanges)

       c. Absent sternocostal head of pectoralis major

   4. Acrocephalosyndactylies

      a. Apert syndrome

         (1) Complete complex syndactyly D2–D4 with common nail, progressive interphalangeal (IP) synostosis of hands and feet, medial deviation of great toe, and tarsal synostosis.

         (2) Craniosynostosis

         (3) Occasional cervical fusions, usually without deformity

      b. Crouzon syndrome

         (1) Craniosynostosis

         (2) Calcaneocuboid coalition, cervical spine fusion

      c. Many other syndromes, such as Saethre-Chotzen, Carpenter

   5. Congenital constriction bands (e.g., Streeter's bands)

      a. A distal (aracral) syndactyly

      b. Thumb rarely involved

      c. Cutaneous rings or amputations

      d. May have distal paresis or deformity (e.g., clubfoot)

B. Polydactyly

   1. Ulnar: frequently isolated, especially in African-American children

   2. Radial: more frequently associated with syndromes, especially radial ray defects

   3. Radial clubhand. This is a spectrum ranging from hypoplasia to complete absence of preaxial parts. It may be isolated or associated with the following conditions.

      a. Blood dyscrasias

         (1) Fanconi's syndrome: anemia to progressive pancytopenia, not present at birth; one-third of patients have renal anomalies; often fatal

         (2) Thrombocytopenia-absent radius (TAR) syndrome: neonatal thrombocytopenia; usually improves with time; frequent knee anomalies

      b. Congenital heart defects. Holt-Oram syndrome: variable cardiac and preaxial deficiency, most commonly atrial septal defect and hypoplastic thumb.

      c. Craniofacial anomalies (Nager syndrome)

      d. Congenital scoliosis

         (1) VATER syndrome (vertebral anomalies, anal atresia, tracheoesophageal fistula (TEF), esophageal atresia, renal and rectal anomalies)

         (2) Goldenhar syndrome (oculo-auriculo-vertebral dysplasia)

         (3) Klippel-Feil syndrome

      e. Implications

         (1) Examine previous chest and abdominal films for vertebral anomalies, or take new radiographs

         (2) Evaluate face, jaw, and palate

         (3) CBC and platelet count

         (4) Ask about feeding (esophageal abnormalities)

         (5) Listen to heart, possibly by echocardiography

         (6) Evaluate genitourinary systems: urinalysis, possibly echocardiography

(7) Perform chromosome analysis if multiple anomalies are found outside of the particular syndrome.
4. Ulnar clubhand: Usually a mild dysgenesis; few frequent associations; may be seen with Cornelia de Lange syndrome
5. Amputated limbs
   a. Single: usually an isolated anomaly but may be associated with idiopathic scoliosis
   b. Congenital ring constriction syndrome: nongenetic, variable rings with two or more of the following findings:
      (1) Grooves in skin, occasionally with lymphatic or vascular impairment
      (2) Transverse amputation with proximal limb normal
      (3) Syndactyly (distal with proximal fenestrations)
      (4) Clubfeet
      (5) Craniofacial defects

XIII. Syndromes due to teratogens
A. Fetal alcohol syndrome
1. Growth disturbance (of both length and weight) through childhood
2. CNS dysfunction and decreased head size; learning deficit or attention deficit disorder or mental retardation
3. Dysmorphic face (mild): (a) small eyes, (b) flat philtrum, (c) thin upper lip
4. Orthopedic features
   a. Contractures (elbows, metacarpophalangeal [MP] and IP joints)
   b. Miscellaneous synostoses
   c. Hip dislocations, clubfeet
   d. Congenital cervical fusion (most often C2–C3)
B. Fetal hydantoin syndrome (due to maternal use of phenytoin)
1. Growth retardation: mild
2. Mental retardation: mild
3. Face: hypertelorism, cleft lip
4. Hands: hypoplasia or absence of phalanges, mostly distal

XIV. Chromosome abnormalities
A. Down syndrome
1. Trisomy, mosaicism, or translocation of chromosome 21
2. Major findings
   a. Mental retardation (variable)
   b. Congenital heart defects: atrioventriculum communis, ventricular septal defect
   c. GI anomalies
   d. Short stature
   e. Leukemia (1%), seizures, diabetes, hypothyroidism (less frequent)
   f. Orthopedic findings
      (1) Delayed walking (age 1½ to 5)
      (2) Ligamentous laxity
      (3) C1–C2 or occiput: C1 laxity (x-ray at about age 4 and yearly if atlanto-dens interval [ADI] >5 mm; fuse if signs of myelopathy exist)
      (4) Scoliosis, idiopathic type
      (5) Hip dislocations: acute, subacute, or habitual
      (6) Slipped capital femoral epiphysis (SCFE)

(7) Perthes disease

(8) Patellar subluxation or dislocation

(9) Metatarsus adductus or hallux valgus

B. Turner syndrome

1. Monosomy X
2. Major findings
   a. Low birth weight and persistent growth retardation
   b. Normal intelligence
   c. Low hairline and webbed neck
   d. Renal and cardiac anomalies, coarctation
   e. Absent or hypoplastic gonads
   f. Orthopedic
      (1) Genu valgum, cubitus valgus
      (2) Scoliosis, idiopathic

C. Noonan syndrome

1. Turner-like phenotype but normal chromosomes
2. Major findings
   a. Mental retardation
   b. Hypertelorism, ptosis, downward-slanting eyes
   c. Increased severity of scoliosis, end-plate changes

D. Klinefelter syndrome

1. Genetics: 47 XXY
2. Clinical features
   a. Asthenic habitus, long legs
   b. Failure of secondary sexual development
   c. Scoliosis
   d. Proximal radioulnar synostosis

E. Cri du chat syndrome

1. Genetics: 5P
2. Clinical findings
   a. Profound mental retardation
   b. Multiple hand and foot anomalies
   c. Scoliosis, congenital

Bibliography

Bethem D, et al. Spinal disorders of dwarfism. *J Bone Joint Surg [Am]* 63:1412, 1981.

Goldberg MJ. *The Dysmorphic Child: An Orthopaedic Perspective.* New York: Raven, 1987.

McKusick V. *Mendelian Inheritance in Man.* Baltimore: Johns Hopkins University Press, 1990.

Morrissey RT. *Lovell & Winter's Pediatric Orthopaedics.* Philadelphia: Lippincott, 1990. Chapters 4, 5, and 6.

Spranger JW, Langer LO, Wiedemann HR. *Bone Dysplasias.* Philadelphia: Saunders, 1974.

Neuromuscular Diseases

Neuromuscular diseases may affect the skeleton due to pathology of the spinal cord or of the peripheral nervous system. These diseases may present with a fully developed clinical picture or with early subtle findings, such as a mild deviation of gait. Tables 4-1 through 4-4 organize the neuromuscular diseases according to the type of neuropathology.

Chapter Outline

I. Evaluation
II. Diseases of the central and peripheral nervous system

I. Evaluation
A. History
1. Prenatal
2. Birth (gestation, weight, Apgar score)
3. Developmental (milestones)
4. Family history

B. Physical examination
1. Motor strength and tone
2. Deep tendon reflexes
3. Cranial nerves
4. Cerebellar signs

C. Serum creatinine phosphokinase (CPK).
Elevation of serum CPK is related to the amount of ongoing muscle necrosis. Serum CPK is abnormal in early and middle phases of Duchenne's and Becker's muscular dystrophies (>20 times normal in childhood and early teens) and in myopathies or myositis. There is minimal to mild elevation of serum CPK in other dystrophies.

D. Dystrophin immunoblot
directly differentiates Duchenne's from Becker's dystrophies and differentiates both from other conditions. Requires small amount of muscle tissue.

E. DNA mutation analysis
requires a small amount of blood or amniotic fluid; it allows prenatal diagnosis.

F. Electromyogram (EMG)
1. Myopathic process: polyphasic low-voltage signal.
2. Neuropathic process: initially, brief biphasic low-voltage fibrillation.
3. Chronic process with reinnervation: prolonged polyphasic fibrillation, increased amplitude.

G. Nerve conduction studies (NCS)
1. Abnormally slowed conduction velocities in conditions involving peripheral nerves only.
2. Normal conduction velocities in spinal muscular atrophy.
3. Normal conduction velocity is 45–65 m/sec for patients over 5 years. Younger children have slower conduction velocity.

H. Muscle biopsy.
Perform biopsy of minimally involved muscle in chronic conditions and of severely involved muscle in acute conditions. Avoid muscles used in EMG testing for 1–2 months. The rectus femoris is used for proximal myopathy, the gastrocnemius for distal. Use light microscopy (store specimens in liquid N_2) for special stains. Evaluate using histologic and histochemical stains.

Stains for type I fibers reveal oxidative metabolism. Type II fibers reveal anaerobic metabolism. The normal ratio of type I to type II fibers is 1:2. Histologic findings are as follows:

1. **Myopathic process**
   a. Necrosis, phagocytosis, and inflammation
   b. Irregularly sized fibers
   c. Type I predominance less than 50%
2. **Neuropathic process**
   a. Small group atrophy
   b. Fiber type grouping, angular fibers
   c. Type II predominance greater than 80%

3. Electron microscopy (glutaraldehyde) is used to differentiate the congenital myopathies with abnormal or absent intracellular structures and to assess glycogen (lipid stores).

I. Nerve biopsy

1. Sural nerve is most commonly biopsied.
2. Guillain-Barré syndrome shows mononuclear infiltrates and focal acute demyelination.
3. Hypertrophic neuropathies show nerve fiber loss, interstitial fibrosis, and "onion bulb" formation.

J. Electrocardiogram (ECG). The ECG is abnormal in Duchenne's muscular dystrophy (sinus tachycardia and right ventricular hypertrophy), Friedreich ataxia, and dystrophia myotonia.

II. Diseases of the central and peripheral nervous system

A. Anterior horn cell diseases are presented in Table 4-1.

B. Other neuropathies are presented in Table 4-2.

C. Muscular dystrophies are presented in Table 4-3.

D. Myotonic disorders are presented in Table 4-4.

Table 4-1. Anterior horn cell diseases

Disease	Age of diagnosis	Inheritance pattern	Life expectancy	Signs	Orthopedic manifestations	Laboratory
Poliomyelitis	Variable	None (infectious)	Related to level of involvement	Asymmetric flaccid paralysis, asymmetric absent DTRs	Contractures, scoliosis	Depends on phase of illness
Spinal muscular atrophy Type I or Werdnig-Hoffmann syndrome	Birth–6 mos	Autosomal recessive gene defect on 5q	Most die in infancy	Marked general weakness, no head control, absent DTR fasciculations, normal sensation	Fractures	Fibrillations at rest; decreased interference pattern; muscle biopsy: atrophic fibers with few hypertrophic fibers
Type II	6–12 mos	Autosomal recessive gene defect on 5q	Early to mid-adulthood	Normal until about 6 mos of age, independent head control in sitting position, never ambulate	Hip subluxation, scoliosis, joint contractures	Normal to slight elevation of CPK; EMG: polyphasic; NCS: normal type II fiber predominance
Type III Kugelberg-Welander	1–2 yrs	Autosomal recessive gene defect on 5q	Over 45 yrs	Normal until about 1 yr of age, ambulate until second decade, then wheelchair; never run or climb stairs	Kyphosis, scoliosis	CPK elevation (50% of patients); EMG: polyphasic, fibrillations; muscle biopsy: atrophic denervated fibers, hypertrophic fibers

DTR = deep tendon reflex; EMG = electromyography; NCS = nerve conduction studies.

Table 4-2. Other central and peripheral neuropathies

	Age of diagnosis	Inheritance pattern	Life expectancy	Signs	Orthopedic manifestations	Laboratory studies
Guillain-Barré syndrome	Variable	None; postviral infection	Approximately 5% mortality	Ascending pain, paresthesia, and weakness	Contractures	↑ CSF protein
Friedreich's ataxia (spinocerebellar degeneration)	Before 10 yrs	Autosomal dominant chromosome 9 defect	<40 yrs	Wide-based gait, weakness, tremor, nystagmus, use wheelchair by age 30, areflexia, cardiomyopathy	Pes cavus, scoliosis	↓↓ Sensory and ↓ motor conduction velocity; abnormal ECG
Hereditary motor and sensory neuropathies						
Type I: Roussy-Levy syndrome or hypertrophic Charcot-Marie-Tooth	Second decade	Autosomal dominant	Normal	Foot deformity, intrinsic wasting, absent reflexes	Equinocavovarus feet, clawing of toes, gait abnormality, hip dysplasia, scoliosis (10%)	↓ Motor conduction velocity
Type II or Charcot-Marie-Tooth disease (neuronal form)	Third to fourth decade	Autosomal dominant	Normal	"Stork legs," foot deformity, distal weakness	Cavus foot deformities, occasional upper extremity intrinsic weakness, gait abnormality	Normal or slowed motor conduction velocity

Table 4-2. *(continued)*

	Age of diagnosis	Inheritance pattern	Life expectancy	Signs	Orthopedic manifestations	Laboratory studies
Type III or Dejerine-Sottas syndrome	Infancy to early childhood	Autosomal recessive	Normal	Foot deformity, footdrop, use wheelchair by fourth decade	Cavus foot, scoliosis	↓↓ Motor conduction velocity, ↑ CSF protein
Type IV or Refsum's disease	Childhood, puberty	Autosomal dominant	Normal	Anosmia, deafness, night blindness, foot deformity, remissions and relapses	Equinocavus feet, scoliosis	↓ Motor conduction velocity, ↑↑ CSF protein, ↑ serum phytanic acid

Table 4-3. Muscular dystrophies

Disease	Age of diagnosis	Inheritance pattern	Abnormal gene	Life expectancy	Signs	Orthopedic manifestations	Laboratory studies
Duchenne's muscular dystrophy	2–6 yrs	X-linked recessive (one-third have new mutation)	Xp21	About 20 yrs	Late walker, calf pseudohypertrophy, Meryon and Gowers's signs and possibly mild mental retardation	Contractures: equinovarus, knee flexion, hip flexion-abduction, wheelchair dependence, scoliosis	↑↑ CPK, ↓↓ dystrophin, EMG: small polyphasic; ECG: abnormal in 80–90%
Becker's muscular dystrophy	Childhood	X-linked recessive	Xp21	Adulthood	Weakness, pseudohypertrophy	Contractures, wheelchair dependence late	↑ CPK, ↓ dystrophin; ECG abnormal 30%
Limb-girdle dystrophy	Second to third decade	Autosomal recessive	—	About 40 yrs	Weakness of pelvic muscles, shoulder muscles, or both	Contractures	↑ CPK, normal dystrophin
Fascioscapulohumeral dystrophy	Second to third decade	Autosomal dominant	4q	Normal	Facial and shoulder girdle weakness, expressionless face	Scapular winging, contractures	Normal CPK, normal dystrophin
Emery-Dreifuss dystrophy (humeroperoneal muscular dystrophy)	2–4 yrs	X-linked recessive	Xq28	Approximately 60 yrs	Muscle weakness, joint contractures	Toe-walking, elbow flexion contractures, neck extension contractures	CPK min ↑, normal dystrophin, ECG: atrioventricular block

Table 4-3. *(continued)*

Disease	Age of diagnosis	Inheritance pattern	Abnormal gene	Life expectancy	Signs	Orthopedic manifestations	Laboratory studies
Congenital myopathies							
Rod-Body myopathy	Variable	—	—	Variable	—	Scoliosis, proximal weakness	—
Central core myopathy	Infancy	—	—	Variable	Nonprogressive	Kyphoscoliosis, equinovarus feet	—
Centronuclear myopathy	Variable	X-linked recessive	Xq28	Variable	—	Developmental hip dysplasia	—

Table 4-4. Myotonic disorders

Disease	Age of diagnosis	Inheritance pattern	Life expectancy	Signs
Mytonia congenita (Thomsen's disease)	0–10 yrs	Autosomal dominant	Normal	Myotonia with initial movement; general muscular hypertrophy; phenytoin and procainamide can decrease myotonia
Paramyotonia congenita (Eulenburg's disease)	Childhood	Autosomal dominant	Normal	Cold-induced episodes of paradoxical myotonia and flaccid paresis associated with K^+ abnormalities treated with quinine or ion exchange resins
Dystrophia myotonia (Steinert's)	Second to third decade	Autosomal dominant	Decreased	Progressive weakness begins distally; gonadal atrophy, cataracts, heart disease, and mental defects associated; develop cervical spine subluxation and wheelchair dependency; endocrine abnormalities
Myotonic dystrophy	Infancy	Autosomal dominant, abnormality on chromosome 9q	Normal	Hypotonia, difficulty swallowing, and expressionless face; develop clubfeet, contractures, and dislocated hips; mental defects and lenticular opacities associated; EMG reveals pathognomonic "dive-bomber" pattern. Disease becomes more severe with second generation.

EMG = electromyography.

Bibliography

Brook, MH. *A Clinician's View of Neuromuscular Diseases* (2nd ed). Baltimore: Williams & Wilkins, 1986.

Shapiro F, Specht L. Current concepts review: The diagnosis and orthopaedic treatment of childhood spinal muscular atrophy, peripheral neuropathy, Friedreich ataxia, and arthrogryposis. *J Bone Joint Surg [Am]* 75:1699, 1993.

Shapiro F, Specht L. Current concepts review: The diagnosis and orthopaedic treatment of inherited muscular diseases of childhood. *J Bone Joint Surg [Am]* 75:439, 1993.

Trauma

Trauma in children can present special treatment problems. This chapter provides basic principles and algorithms both for isolated fractures and for polytrauma in children. Common diaphyseal fractures are not covered if there are no unique pediatric features. A bibliography is provided at the end of each section for further information.

Chapter Outline

I. Basic principles
A. Physeal fractures
1. Classification
  a. There are many classification systems for physeal fractures, including those of Aitken, Ogden, Salter, and Peterson. Their goals are (1) to facilitate communication, (2) to predict the risk of growth disturbance, and (3) to help determine treatment.
  b. The classifications provide information on the following:
  (1) Physeal alignment
  (2) Articular alignment
  (3) Stability and risk of displacement
  c. Classifications generally predict the risk of growth disturbance, with some notable exceptions—the distal femur and the distal tibia—where there is a high risk of growth disturbance even in the "benign" fracture types, such as Salter I and II. This may be due to the complex physeal anatomy as well as to the compressive forces involved.
  d. The **Salter classification** is the most widely used system (Fig. 5-1). Note that type V fractures are rarely seen.
  e. The Peterson classification recognizes a broader spectrum of injuries than other classifications.
B. Management of the polytrauma patient
1. Definition
  The polytrauma patient has more than one organ system injured or more than one component affected within one organ system.
  a. Laboratory studies. CBC, blood type and cross, urinalysis, BUN, creatinine clearance, amylase, and electrolytes as indicated.
  b. Indications for radiographic studies
  (1) Cervical, thoracic, or lumbar spine
    (a) Tender
    (b) Unconscious
    (c) Neurologically abnormal
  (2) Pelvis
    (a) Tender
    (b) Unconscious
    (c) Hematuria present
  (3) Skull
    (a) Head trauma and loss of consciousness longer than 5 minutes; hematoma
    (b) Skull depression
    (c) Focal neurologic signs
    (d) Cerebrospinal fluid from nose or middle ear
    (e) Blood in middle ear
  (4) CT of head
    (a) A score on the Glasgow coma score less than 8 (see section 4, below).
    (b) Focal neurologic signs
  (5) CT of abdomen
    (a) Shock
    (b) Severe head injury
    (c) Abnormal abdominal examination

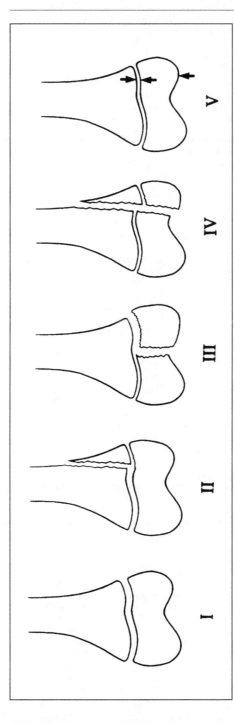

Fig. 5-1. Salter-Harris classification of physeal injuries. Type I: fracture purely across physis. Type II: fracture across physis and metaphysis. Type III: fracture across part of physis and epiphysis. Type IV: fracture across metaphysis, physis, and epiphysis. Type V: crush injury (arrows) without fracture. (Reproduced with permission from HA Peterson. Physeal fractures. *J Pediatr Orthop* 14:442, 1994.)

2. Initial evaluation

a. Physical examination

(1) Primary survey to detect most urgent priorities (ABCDE).

A   Airway
B   Breathing (ventilation)
C   Circulation (hemorrhage)
D   Disability (neurologic status)
E   Exposure (temperature)

(2) Secondary survey
(a) Complete physical examination
(b) History of event
(c) Personal medical history
(d) Laboratory and x-ray results
(e) Re-evaluation and stabilization

3. Normal vital signs for children (Table 5-1)

4. Glasgow coma score

	Response	**Score**
Eye opening	None	1
	To pain	2
	To voice	3
	Spontaneous	4
Verbal	None	1
	Incomprehensible	2
	Inappropriate	3
	Disoriented	4
	Oriented	5
Motor	None	1
	Decerebrate	2
	Decorticate	3
	Withdraws to pain	4
	Localizes pain	5
	Obeys	6
Total	Up to 15 points	

5. Adjuncts in management

a. Intracranial pressure measurement indications

(1) Glasgow coma scale score under 5, or under 8 if shock present.
(2) CT scan showing mass or shift.
(3) Progressive neurologic deterioration.

Table 5-1. Normal vital signs for children

Age	Pulse (beats/min)	Respirations (per min)	Blood pressure (mm S/D)
1–6 mos	130 ± 45	30–40	80/46
6–12 mos	114 ± 40	24–30	95/65
1–2 yrs	110 ± 40	20–30	99/65
2–6 yrs	105 ± 35	20–25	100/60
6–12 yrs	95 ± 30	16–20	110/60
12 yrs	80 ± 25	12–16	120/60

    b. Parenteral nutrition is indicated in the polytrauma patient if enteral feeding is not expected within 24 hours.
    c. Repeat **physical examination** should be performed at 24 and 48 hours due to the incidence of missed injuries. Bone scan is an alternative.
    d. Deep venous thrombosis prophylaxis indications in polytrauma
      (1) Oral contraceptive use
      (2) Vascular injury
      (3) Sickle cell anemia
      (4) Prolonged immobility in older adolescent

II. Shoulder injuries

A. Principles

1. The **proximal humeral physis** is one of the most active in the skeleton. It gives rise to 80% of the length of humerus; therefore it has tremendous potential to remodel deformity.
2. Ossification begins at 6 months in the proximal humeral epiphysis and ceases at age 15 (females) and 17 (males). The center for the greater tuberosity appears at 1 year. The medial clavicle physis closes at approximately age 23.

B. Birth fractures

1. Risk factors
   a. Difficult delivery
   b. Large size
   c. Breech presentation
2. Presentation
   a. Pseudoparalysis
   b. Rule out sepsis and brachial plexus injury
3. Diagnosis: plain x-rays or ultrasound.
4. Treatment: wrap with elastic bandage with arm to chest for 2 weeks.

C. Proximal humeral fractures

1. **Background**
   a. Preadolescent: usually fracture of metaphyseal region.
   b. Adolescent: physeal fracture; Salter II or I.
   c. Mechanism: axial load or abduction-external rotation.
   d. Muscle insertions with respect to physis: Internal and external rotators all on proximal fragment; deltoid and pectoralis on the distal fragment. Distal fragment usually displaces anteriorly and laterally.
2. **Criteria for acceptable alignment**
   a. Child under age 12: Virtually any alignment is acceptable.
   b. Child over age 12: Shortening or overlap (in upright position) should be less than 3 cm, angulation less than 45 degrees.
3. **Classification of displacement** (pediatric) (Neer and Horowitz)

I	< 5 mm translation
II	5 mm–33%
II	33–66%
V	> 66%

Most displacements are grade IV. Translation itself is not a problem.

Note: The appearance of the fracture on radiographic film is not the same as its appearance later in sling. Angulation usually improves when limb is upright.

4. Treatment methods
   a. Sling
   b. Traction
   c. Shoulder spica
   d. Abduction brace
   e. Internal fixation

5. Results
   a. No randomized studies of treatment methods exist.
   b. Beringer and colleagues (1993) at Akron Children's Hospital conducted a 9-year follow-up study of 46 patients with severe displacement. At final follow-up there was no difference between operative and non-operative groups despite imperfect anatomic results in some nonoperative patients. Complications occurred in three of nine operative patients.
   c. Baxter and Willey followed 57 patients for 2 years or more after closed treatment. Maximum residual shortening was 2 cm, regardless of treatment, and angulation was insignificant.

6. Treatment recommendations
   a. Sling and swathe as long as any growth remains.
   b. Closed or open reduction with internal fixation (CRIF or ORIF) under the following conditions:
      (1) Severe head injury with spasticity.
      (2) In cases of polytrauma—to facilitate management.
      (3) Vascular injury.
      (4) Tenting skin with risk of breakdown.

7. Unicameral bone cyst (UBC)
   a. Common cause of proximal humerus fracture in children.
   b. Differential diagnosis
      (1) Eosinophilic granuloma
      (2) Aneurysmal bone cyst (ABC)
      (3) Fibrous dysplasia
      (4) Fibrous cortical defect
      (5) Telangiectatic osteosarcoma
   c. Treatment
      (1) Sling to heal fracture for 4–6 weeks.
      (2) Cyst regresses in approximately 20% of patients.
      (3) Assess and discuss risk of refracture with family: It depends mainly on cortical thickness.
      (4) Inject with methylprednisolone or bone graft substance if:
         (a) Persistent thin cortex
         (b) High desired activity level
         (c) Family prefers active treatment
      (5) Several injections may be required.

D. Sternoclavicular injuries
   1. Medial clavicle is the last epiphysis to appear and to close (about age 23).
   2. Provides 80% of clavicle growth.

3. Injury may be a dislocation or a fracture.
4. CT scan provides most accurate visualization if diagnosis is unclear.
5. Signs of **significant** displacement
   a. Venous congestion
   b. Decreased pulse
   c. Difficulty breathing or swallowing
   d. Sensation of choking
6. Treatment
   a. Anterior displacement usually requires no treatment.
   b. Posterior displacement: Treat if there are significant symptoms.
   c. Closed reduction; may use towel clips.
   d. No internal fixation; use sutures if unstable.

Bibliography

Baxter MP, Willey JJ. Fractures of the proximal humerus. *J Bone Joint Surg [Br]* 68:570, 1986.

MacEwen GD, Kasser JR, Heinrich S. *Pediatric Fractures.* Baltimore: Williams & Wilkins, 1993.

Neer CS, Horowitz BS. Fractures of the proximal humeral epiphyseal plate. *Clin Orthop* 41:24, 1965.

III. Elbow injuries
A. Lateral condyle fracture
1. **Background**
   a. Vascular supply to the capitellum and lateral trochlea enters posteriorly.
   b. Fracture may occur with varus or valgus force.
   c. Distinguish this injury from a transphyseal separation by lack of swelling and tenderness medially and by normal alignment of humerus with forearm (Fig. 5-2B); ultrasound may help.
   d. Oblique x-rays may show fracture line best.
2. **Principles**
   a. This is one of the few pediatric fractures in which nonunion may occur (5–10%).
   b. Cast is rarely able to maintain reduction of a displaced lateral condylar fragment.
3. **Treatment recommendations**
   a. If displacement is less than 2 mm, splint in 90–100 degrees flexion and pronation. Recheck at 5 days and 10 days. ORIF if further displacement.
   b. If displacement is 2 mm or greater *or* follow-up is unreliable, attempt closed reduction (optional).
      (1) If reduced, then fix internally.
      (2) If not reduced, then ORIF.
      (3) Avoid posterior dissection: Visualize reduction anteriorly.
      (4) For internal fixation: Two divergent pins are preferred; these may cross the physis if necessary. Use metaphyseal screw if metaphyseal fragment is large.

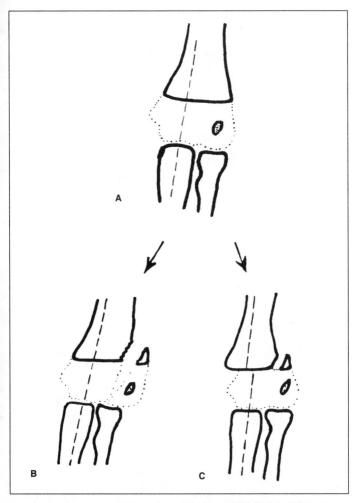

Fig. 5-2. Differentiation of lateral condyle from distal humeral physeal
Salter II fracture. In the latter, displacement of the entire forearm follows
the metaphyseal fragment. In minimally displaced fractures, physical
examination, ultrasound, arthrogram, or MRI may be helpful. A. Normal
alignment of ulna and humerus. B. Alignment maintained in lateral
condyle fracture. C. Alignment lost in distal humeral Salter II physeal
fractures.

> (5) Usually remove pins and splint at 6–8 weeks
>   post-operation.
> 4. **Fiberglass** allows best visualization of fracture. Follow
>   patient at least until union is clearly evident.
> 5. **Late presentation** (displaced and nonunited for more
>   than 6 wks)
>   a. Approach anteriorly with graft and internal fixation
>   if in good position (early). After 3 weeks, operate only

for symptoms of lateral instability. Avoid excessive dissection.

  b. Valgus osteotomy if significant deformity exists.

  c. Ulnar nerve anterior transposition if deformity is increasing.

B. Medial epicondyle fractures

1. Background

  a. Medial epicondyle begins to ossify at age 4–6 and fuses at approximately age 15.

  b. This fracture is most common in ages 9–12, and is more common in males than females.

  c. Significance

  (1) Medial collateral ligament of the ulna attaches to the base of the epicondyle.

  (2) Entrapped medial epicondyle in the joint is occasionally missed.

  (3) Consider medial *condylar* extension in patients under age 9 with large metaphyseal fragment.

2. Treatment

  a. Principle: Some displacement is well tolerated unless forceful loading is anticipated.

  b. Indications for ORIF

  (1) Epicondyle in joint despite attempt at manipulation.

  (2) High valgus stresses are anticipated (e.g., in the dominant arm of throwing athlete) in the patient with a displaced epicondyle. Stress test in 15-degree flexion may be of interest, but no specific guidelines for interpretation of this test exist.

  c. Technique of ORIF. Exposure is easier in prone position; use screw or percutaneous pin; ulnar nerve transposition is not recommended in most patients.

  d. Indications for closed reduction. All cases not meeting the criteria for ORIF in part **b** above, including the following special cases:

  (1) Acute ulnar neuropathy. This is likely to resolve with time. It is not a specific indication for ORIF or ulnar nerve transposition.

  (2) Displacement greater than 5 mm but not intraarticular.

  (3) Epicondyle fracture with elbow dislocation.

C. Elbow dislocations

1. Background

  a. These occur mainly in teenagers and adults.

  b. Before skeletal maturity, approximately 60% have associated fracture of the medial epicondyle, proximal radius, coronoid process, or olecranon.

  c. Open dislocations have a high incidence of arterial injury.

2. Treatment

  a. Carefully examine for associated fractures, especially those of the radial head or lateral condyle; these may alter treatment plan.

  b. Closed reduction with sedation or anesthesia is successful in most cases.

  c. Instruct parent in vascular examination or admit overnight if questionable.

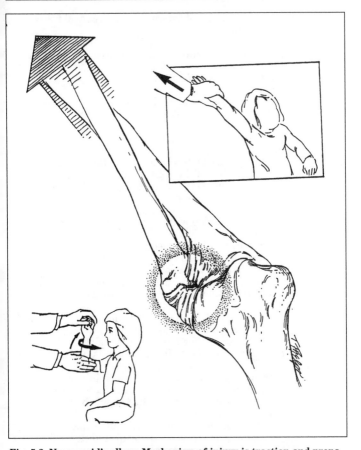

Fig. 5-3. Nursemaid's elbow. Mechanism of injury is traction and pronation (upper right). Pathology is partial infolding of annular ligament of
radial head (center). Reduction is by flexion and supination (lower
left). (Reproduced with permission from FA Oski. *Principles and
Practices of Pediatrics* [2nd ed]. Philadelphia: Lippincott, 1994. P 1037.)

       d. Splint for 2–3 weeks.

       e. Follow up to rule out posterolateral instability.

       f. If dislocation is missed for longer than 1 week, open
reduction will be necessary, but this gives satisfactory results in children even months after dislocation.

D. Nursemaid's elbow (annular ligament entrapment)

    1. Injury caused by longitudinal traction in child aged 1–4.

    2. Elbow held slightly flexed, pronated, and guarded.

    3. Treatment: Flex and supinate (Fig. 5-3, lower left).
Immobilization is usually unnecessary unless recurrent.

E. Radial head and neck fractures

    1. Background

       a. Ossification develops around ages 4–5 in proximal
radial epiphysis.

   b. Much of the radial neck is intracapsular.
   c. Wilkins classification
      (1) Primary displacement of **radial head**
         (a) Valgus fractures
         (b) Salter I and II
         (c) Salter IV
         (d) Metaphyseal
         (e) Fractures with elbow dislocation (reduction injuries)
         (f) Dislocation injuries
      (2) Primary dislocation of **radial neck** (e.g., Monteggia variant)

2. Treatment guidelines
   a. If angulation is less than 30 degrees, accept as is; begin range of motion in 1–2 weeks
   b. If angulation is 30–45 degrees, manipulate, but accept closed result.
   c. If angulation is greater than 45 degrees (approximately) or translocated, manipulate, but perform ORIF if unsuccessful.

3. Manipulation techniques (under anesthesia)
   a. Patterson technique involves traction in extension. Use fluoroscopy to profile fracture. Press on displaced fragment while applying varus stress to forearm.
   b. Flexion-pronation technique: Flex elbow 90 degrees. Rotate forearm from full supination to pronation while applying pressure anteriorly to radial head.
   c. Percutaneous leverage via Kirschner wire with elbow in extension. Use fluoroscopy. Push the radial head back into place with a K wire. Pin starts proximally in the "corner" of the radial head, behind the posterior interosseous nerve.

4. Maintaining reduction
   a. Flexion to 90 degrees is satisfactory for many cases.
   b. For unstable fractures, oblique Kirschner wire from proximal to distal fragment is preferable. The K wire crosses the fracture but not the joint. Protect with posterior splint.

F. Monteggia fracture-dislocation
   1. Principle. Radial head dislocates in the direction of a line drawn through the distal ulnar fragment. Even a slight ulnar bow may signal radial head subluxation (Fig. 5-4B).
   2. Classification (based on direction of radial head dislocation)
      a. Anterior
      b. Posterior
      c. Lateral
      d. Anterior with fracture of proximal third of the radius
   3. Treatment
      a. Reduction mechanism is basically that used to reduce the ulnar fracture, with supination added for anterior and lateral types of dislocation.
      b. Failure to achieve or maintain radial head reduction should lead to intramedullary pinning or plating of the ulna.

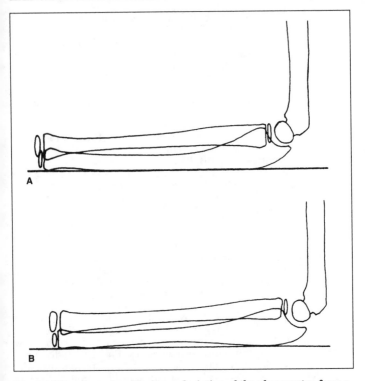

Fig. 5-4. Ulnar bow sign. Maximum deviation of the ulnar cortex from a straight line should be 1 mm (A). If greater (B), it should suggest plastic deformation of the ulna and possible radial head subluxation, a subtle example of which is shown in B. (Reproduced with permission from TL Lincoln, SJ Mubarak. "Isolated" radial head dislocation. *J Pediatr Orthop* 14:455, 1994.)

        c. If intramedullary pinning or plating of the ulna does not reduce the radial head, openly reduce it
    4. Late-presenting Monteggia fracture-dislocation can be operatively reduced up to 2 years after injury. Correct the ulnar bow and reconstruct the annular ligament (Bell Tawse procedure).

G. Supracondylar humerus fractures
  1. Classification
    a. Direction of displacement
      (1) Most such fractures are due to hyperextension (periosteal hinge is posterior).
      (2) Few of these fractures are due to flexion (periosteal hinge is anterior).
    b. Degree of displacement

      Type I: Undisplaced
      Type II (hinged or greenstick): Intact posterior cortex
      Type III: Completely displaced

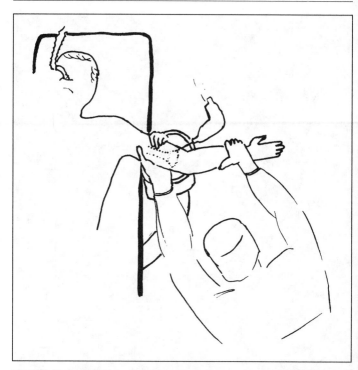

Fig. 5-5. One technique of closed reduction and percutaneous pinning of supracondylar fracture. Longitudinal traction is applied in slight flexion to correct angulation yet allow visualization. Fluoroscope receiver serves as platform.

2. **Principle.** Type III fractures produce an appreciable incidence of nerve and artery damage. They have little intrinsic stability. Therefore, the best results in type III occur with reduction and pin fixation. Carefully document status of all nerves and circulation before treatment.
3. **Treatment**
   a. **Type II.** Correct hyperextension and any angulation. Flex greater than 90 degrees. Pin if needed to maintain reduction.
   b. **Type III**
      (1) Attempt closed reduction by correction of translation, angulation, and hyperextension. Maintain reduction by longitudinal traction in slight flexion. Carry out percutaneous pin fixation (Fig. 5-5) with one medial and one lateral pin or two lateral pins. Both pins should start distal to fracture site. Lateral pin should engage a portion of capitellum; medial pin should be slightly medial and anterior on epicondyle to avoid ulnar nerve (Fig. 5-6). Make a small incision to clear a track. The lateral pin is at about 30

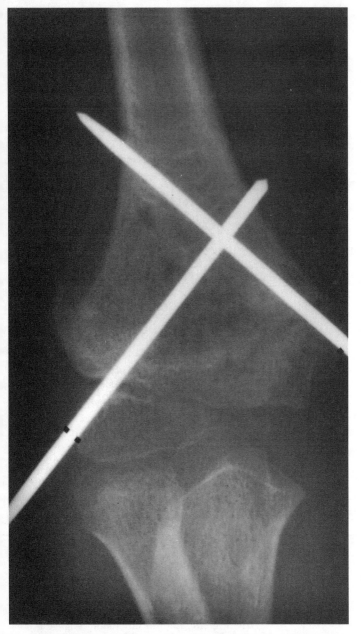

Fig. 5-6. Desired pin placement for medial and lateral pin technique in supracondylar fracture.

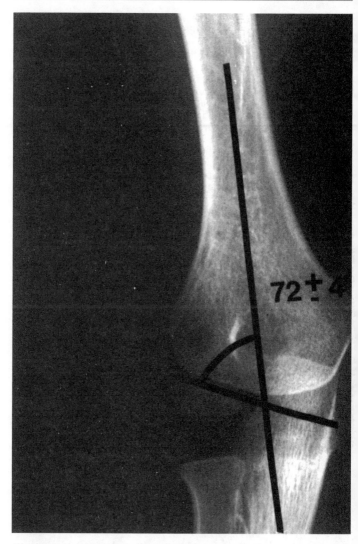

Fig. 5-7. Baumann angle measurement and its normal range.

degrees to the long axis of the humerus; the medial pin is at 45 degrees.

(2) If anatomic closed reduction is not possible, perform open reduction. Check alignment of fracture using the Baumann angle (Fig. 5-7). Normal is 72 ±4 degrees.

(3) Aftercare. Begin supervised range of motion exercises at about 3 weeks with temporary splint removal. Remove pins at 6 weeks.

4. **Nerve injury**
   a. **Frequency.** Radial > median > anterior interosseous > ulnar.
   b. **Treatment.** If deficit is present before reduction, it is probably a neuropraxia due to the injury; proceed with closed reduction. If there is no return of function by 5 months after injury, obtain electromyogram; explore and perform neurolysis if recovery does not take place.
5. **Arterial insufficiency**
   a. Reduce fracture; do not hyperflex. If perfusion returns, pin fracture. If perfusion does not return, perform open exploration through anterior Henry approach.
      (1) If artery is entrapped, release and watch.
      (2) If the artery is in spasm, use topical lidocaine.
      (3) If there is an intimal tear, repair, or resect and graft.
      (4) If the artery is transected, perform a vein graft.
   b. Measure compartment pressures after reperfusion, and perform fasciotomy if needed.

Bibliography

General

Wilkins KE. Elbow Fractures. In C Rockwood, KE Wilkins, JH Beaty (eds), *Fractures in Children.* New York: Lippincott, 1996.

Lateral Condyle Fracture

Badelon O et al. Lateral humeral condyle fractures in children. *J Pediatr Orthop* 8:31, 1988.

Flynn JC. Nonunion of slightly displaced fractures of the lateral humeral condyle in children: An update. *J Pediatr Orthop* 9:691, 1989.

Foster DF et al. Lateral humeral condyle fractures in children. *J Pediatr Orthop* 5:16, 1985.

Medial Epicondyle Fracture

Josefsson PO, Danielsson LG. Epicondylar elbow fracture in children: 35-year follow-up of 56 unreduced cases. *Acta Orthop Scand* 57:313, 1986.

Elbow Dislocation

Carlioz H, Abbes Y. Posterior dislocation of the elbow in children. *J Pediatr Orthop* 4:8, 1984.

Fowles JV et al. Untreated posterior dislocation of the elbow in children. *J Bone Joint Surg [Am]* 66:921, 1984.

Nestor BJ et al. Ligamentous reconstruction for posterolateral rotatory instability of the elbow. *J Bone Joint Surg [Am]* 74:1235, 1992.

Radial Head and Neck Fractures

Metaizeau JP et al. Reduction and fixation of displaced radial neck fractures by closed intramedullary pinning. *J Pediatr Orthop* 13:355, 1993.

Steele JA, Graham HK. Angulated radial neck fractures in children. *J Bone Joint Surg [Am]* 74:761, 1992.

Olecranon Fractures

Dormans JP, Rang M. Fractures of the olecranon and radial neck in children. *Orthop Clin North Am* 21:2257, 1990.

Supracondylar Fractures

Culp RW et al. Neural injuries associated with supracondylar fractures of the humerus in children. *J Bone Joint Surg [Am]* 72:1211, 1990.

Pirone AM, Graham HK, Krajbich JI. Management of displaced extension-type supracondylar fractures of the humerus in children. *J Bone Joint Surg [Am]* 70:641,1988.

IV. Hand and wrist injuries
A. Hand injuries
1. **Distal phalanx fractures.** Pediatric mallet finger is the most common serious fracture of this bone. It is often an open injury. Treatment consists of the following:
   a. Replace nail under fold.
   b. CRIF or ORIF fracture as indicated.
   c. Follow to rule out infection.
2. **Phalangeal neck** (subcondylar) fractures
   a. Principles
      (1) Most occur in proximal phalanx.
      (2) Volar angulation is the most common type.
      (3) Minimal remodeling occurs in this region.
   b. Treatment of displaced fracture
      (1) Closed reduction
      (2) Transarticular percutaneous pinning for 3 weeks
      (3) Buddy-tape for 1 week
      (4) Late presentation: may openly reconstruct up to 4 weeks after fracture.
   c. Malunion. Loss of flexion may occur if malposition with bony impingement is allowed to persist. Treatment consists of a volar approach and removal of bony block to flexion.
3. **Phalangeal shaft fractures**
   a. Less common in children than adults
   b. May accept 10 degrees dorsal or palmar angulation
   c. Treatment: Immobilize with short arm cast or splint
4. **Metacarpophalangeal joint injuries**
   a. The collateral ligament does not protect the physis of the proximal phalanx or the metacarpal head.
   b. "Extra octave" fracture of small finger (Salter I or II with abducted position)
      (1) Reduce using a pencil in the web space as a fulcrum.
      (2) Reduction should be maintained when pressure is released.
      (3) Hold with rolled cotton gauze between digits.
   c. Intraarticular fractures
      (1) If fragment is greater than 25% of joint surface or involves any tendon insertion, it must be reduced to within 2 mm of anatomic position.
      (2) Growth arrest is seen in less than 1% of patients.
   d. Dislocation
      (1) Simple metacarpaphalangeal joint dislocation is

the most common type. However, complex (irreducible) dorsal dislocation also occurs often. The essential features of this type are:
- **(a)** Volar plate entrapped
- **(b)** Joint space wide, but finger looks nearly straight
- **(c)** Sesamoids interposed
- **(d)** Skin dimpled on volar surface
- **(2)** Treatment
  - **(a)** Make one or two attempts at closed reduction
  - **(b)** Open reduction: From volar or dorsal approach, incise superficial transverse ligament lateral to volar plate, remove volar plate from joint, and reduce fracture

5. **Pediatric thumb metacarpal fractures**
- **a.** Metaphyseal or Salter I and II fractures. Treatment consists of attempting closed reduction and cast; pin if unacceptable.
- **b.** Pediatric Bennett's fractures. Treatment consists of closed reduction or ORIF if displacement exceeds 1 mm.
- **c.** Gamekeeper's fracture (ulnar collateral ligament avulsion). Stener lesion, consisting of the ulnar corner of the epiphysis of the proximal phalanx, usually indicates a Salter III type. Treatment consists of ORIF if displaced more than 1 mm or if x-rays show no fracture but there is a positive stress test at 45 degrees of flexion. This indicates ligamentous tear, possibly entrapped under the adductor.

6. **Scaphoid fractures**
- **a.** Much less frequent in children than adults
- **b.** May occur with distal radius fracture
- **c.** If diagnosed within 3 months, fracture usually heals with a short arm-thumb spica cast
- **d.** If union is delayed longer than 3 months, a bone graft will be required.

B. **Distal radial physeal fractures**
1. Salter I and II are the most common types.
2. Perform one or two gentle reductions with adequate analgesia or anesthesia if necessary.
3. Immobilize in neutral position or pronation.
4. Growth arrest is rare.
5. Complications
   - **a.** Compartment syndrome
   - **b.** Median nerve injury

Bibliography

Crick JC, Franco RS, Conners JJ. Fractures about the IP joints in children. *J Orthop Trauma* 1:318, 1988.

Simmons BP, Peter TT. Subcondylar fossa reconstruction. *J Hand Surg [Am]* 12:1079, 1982.

V. Spine injuries
  A. Cervical spine
   1. General principles
     a. Child should be transported on special backboard with recess under head to accommodate large head, or lift under shoulders.
     b. Obtain x-rays if:
       (1) Unconscious patient
       (2) Neck pain
       (3) Head or facial bruising
     c. Recommended radiographs
       (1) Lateral, anteroposterior, open mouth.
       (2) Oblique x-rays only if dislocation or subluxation is suspected.
     d. Normal values. See Chapter 1, sec. **I**, Figure 1-11 for radiographic normal values of the cervical spine in children. Also refer to this section for normal ossification patterns.
   2. Odontoid fracture. Reduce and hold in halo or Minerva cast for 8 weeks, then in Philadelphia collar for 4 weeks.
   3. Atlas (C1) fracture (Jefferson fracture)
     a. Minimum (<7 mm) spread of lateral masses: Hold in Philadelphia collar.
     b. If significant spread of lateral masses (>7 mm) is seen, then treat with traction for 4 weeks followed by collar.
   4. C1–C2 rotatory subluxation
     a. CT scan is the best study to confirm diagnosis.
     b. Symptom duration less than 1 week: Treat with collar, analgesics, bed rest, and exercises to reduce subluxation.
     c. Symptom duration longer than 1 week: Treat with halter traction and exercises.
     d. Symptom duration longer than 1 month: Treat with halo-gravity traction, attempting reduction. Fuse in situ if not reducible.
   5. Transverse ligament insufficiency or os odontoideum. Assess with flexion-extension views.
     a. Atlanto-dens interval (distance between arch of C1 and odontoid) less than 4 mm is normal.
     b. If the interval is 4–8 mm, treat with collar, restrict activities.
     c. If the interval is greater than 8 mm or any neurologic abnormalities exist, perform posterior fusion of C1–C2.
   6. C2 pedicle fracture (hangman's fracture).
     a. If C2–C3 disc is intact, immobilize in collar or halo vest.
     b. If C2–C3 disc is disrupted, consider anterior C2–C3 spine fusion.
  B. Thoracic and lumbar spine
   1. Compression fracture
     a. If vertebral body collapse is less than 20%, mobilize as tolerated.
     b. If collapse is 20% or greater, provide thoraco-lumbo-sacral orthosis (TLSO) for comfort; mobilize as tolerated.
   2. Burst fractures
     a. If patient is neurologically normal, immobilize with

cast for 6–8 weeks, then mobilize as tolerated. Open reduction and internal stabilization is an option if deformity is great but criteria are not agreed on.

  b. If neurologic deficit is present, consider decompression anteriorly or posteriorly and fuse.

3. Flexion-distraction (Chance) injuries

  a. Attempt reduction in extension, and immobilize for 6–8 weeks.

  b. If reduction is not obtained or is still unstable, then openly reduce and internally fix.

VI. Femoral shaft fractures

A. Principles

1. Mechanism: Pedestrian struck by car (most common); fall or sports injury (less common); passenger in motor vehicle accident (least common).

2. Acceptable reduction consists of a final varus or valgus angle of up to 10 degrees, anterior or posterior bow of up to 20 degrees, and shortening of up to 2.5 cm.

3. Overgrowth of approximately 1 cm occurs between ages 2 and 10.

4. Family factors are important in choosing treatment.

5. Consider child abuse if patient is under age 2.

6. Hip spica cast is not a good way to maintain length if the fracture has significant overlap.

B. Treatment

1. Age less than 6. If resting overlap is less than 2 cm or telescope test shows less than 3-cm shortening, immobilize with spica cast. If not, immobilize with traction (in hospital or at home), pin-in-plaster cast, or external fixator.

2. Age 6–10

  a. If resting overlap is less than 2 cm or telescope test shows less than 3 cm shortening, spica cast is an option, if parents desire.

  b. Preferred options: external fixator, flexible intramedullary rods or plate, or traction in hospital or at home.

3. Older than age 10

  a. Intramedullary rod, with careful preparation of entry hole to avoid disrupting vessels at femoral neck.

  b. External fixator

  c. Plate

C. Time to union (mean)

Infant	≤ 4 weeks
Age 2–4	6 weeks
Age 4–6	8 weeks
Age 6–8	10 weeks

Times are longer for open or high-energy injuries, shorter for patients with significant closed head injuries.

D. Subtrochanteric fractures

1. Overgrowth also occurs here as in the shaft: 1 cm on the average.

2. Angulation of 25 degrees in any plane is acceptable.

3. Fracture tends to develop anterior bow.

4. Fracture is harder to image by plain films in a cast.

5. Treatment
  a. Traction for 3 weeks in 90-degree flexion, then spica cast in the same position, or
  b. ORIF with plate
  c. External fixator

VII. Physeal injuries about the knee
A. Normal anatomy and growth
  1. The length of the lower limbs doubles between age 4 and maturity.
  2. Features of the distal femoral physis
    a. Quadripodal.
    b. Ligaments concentrate stress on this physis.
    c. Growth is 1 cm/year until age 13½ (girls), age 15½ (boys).
    d. The blood supply to the physis primarily comes from epiphyseal vessels, with some contribution from periosteal vessels.
  3. Features of the proximal tibial physis
    a. An anterior extension continues down to the tubercle.
    b. Ligaments, fibula, and semimembranosus insertion protect physis.
    c. Growth is 8 mm/year.

B. Distal femoral physeal fracture
  1. Most common physeal injury about the knee.
  2. Mechanism
    a. Hyperextension, or
    b. Valgus force
  3. Findings
    a. Hemarthrosis, especially in Salter III and IV
    b. May be missed in polytrauma patient
    c. Ligamentous injury may coexist
  4. Radiographs
    a. AP, lateral with oblique and tunnel views if needed.
    b. Stress view if occult fracture suspected.
    c. Plain tomograms or CT scan for complex Salter III and IV if fracture pattern or displacement is in question.
    d. Obtain arteriogram:
      (1) If vascular examination is abnormal.
      (2) If proximal tibia physis is fractured and significantly posteriorly displaced.
      (3) Incidence of vascular injury is less than 1%.
        In most cases, arteriogram is not necessary, especially in varus-valgus injuries. Instead, check circulation before and after reduction and instruct nurses in monitoring it.
  5. Treatment
    a. Gentle closed reduction.
    b. Five degrees varus or valgus angle is the maximum acceptable in Salter types I and II.
    c. Open reduction if irreducible by closed methods.
    d. Pin if unstable.
    e. ORIF all displaced Salter type IV fractures.
    f. Assure physeal alignment by direct inspection at fracture and periphery as well as fluoroscopy.
    g. Immobilization
      (1) Long leg cast if limb is slender and fracture is stable

(2) Spica cast otherwise
h. Begin range of motion exercises by 6 weeks.
i. Follow up for at least 1 year to rule out growth plate injury.

6. **Results**
   a. Twenty-five to 50% of patients have length discrepancy greater than 1 cm.
   b. Twenty-five percent of patients have angular deformity greater than 5 degrees.

7. **Treatment of physeal bridge**
   a. **Imaging**
      (1) Growth lines visible on plain film should be present and parallel to physis by 4–6 months if growth is normal.
      (2) Tomograms (plain, not CT scan) if bridge is suspected.
      (3) MRI. Discuss with radiologist before study. It is currently the preferred study.
   b. **Indications for resection**
      (1) Area of bar less than 50% of physeal area.
      (2) More than 2 years of growth remaining.

C. **Proximal tibial physis injury**
   1. Twenty-five percent as common as distal femur physeal injury; 5% have popliteal or peroneal injuries.
   2. **Mechanisms**
      a. Hyperextension
      b. Valgus injury
      c. Fifty percent occur in sports
   3. **Treatment**
      a. Closed or open reduction based on standard criteria
      b. Close vascular monitoring

D. **Tibial tubercle fractures**
   1. **Background**
      a. Some patients have a prior history of an Osgood-Schlatter lesion.
      b. Frequency in males is much greater than in females
      c. Usual age range is 14–16
      d. Almost always occur in jumping sports
   2. **Treatment**
      a. Closed reduction if minimally displaced and patient can actively extend knee
      b. **ORIF**
         (1) Clear bed of interposed tissue.
         (2) Use screw if there is a large fragment and patient is near maturity.
         (3) Otherwise, suture tendon and periosteum.
   3. **Complications (rare)**
      a. Recurvatum: only if very young (<age 11)
      b. Loss of flexion

Bibliography

Burkhart SS, Peterson HA. Fractures of the proximal tibial epiphysis. *J Bone Joint Surg [Am]* 61:996, 1979.

Christie JF, Dvonch V. Tibial tuberosity avulsion fracture in adolescents. *J Pediatr Orthop* 1:391, 1991.

Ogden JA, Trass RB, Murphy MJ. Fractures of the tibial tuberosity in adolescents. *J Bone Joint Surg [Am]* 62:205, 1980.

Riseborough EJ, Barrett IR, Shapiro F. Growth disturbances following distal femoral physeal fracture-separation. *J Bone Joint Surg [Am]* 65:855, 1983.

Williamson RV, Staheli LT. Partial physeal growth arrest: Treatment by bridge resection and fat interposition. *J Pediatr Orthop* 10:769, 1990.

VIII. Physeal injuries about the ankle

A. Background. Normal growth

1. Distal tibial and fibular epiphyses appear at approximately age 2 and close at age 15–16.
2. Anterolateral portion closes last.
3. Distal fibular physis is normally at the level of tibial joint surface.

B. Fracture classification (Dias)

1. Supination-external rotation (SER)
2. Pronation-external rotation (PER)
3. Supination-plantar flexion (SPF)
4. Supination-inversion (SI)
5. Axial loading
6. Tillaux
7. Triplane

C. Nonarticular physeal fractures

1. Closed or open reduction, depending on standard criteria (5 degrees varus or valgus angle is acceptable).
2. Check rotation by x-ray and clinically by thigh-foot angle.
3. If displaced, use long leg cast in most cases.

D. Tillaux fractures

1. Avulsion of anterolateral corner of distal tibial epiphysis. Anterior inferior tibiofibular ligament avulses unfused epiphyseal fragment. Usually occurs near maturity.
2. **Mechanism of injury:** Supination-external rotation.
3. **Treatment.** Reduce with internal rotation. If gap persists greater than 2 mm, then ORIF.

E. Triplane fractures. Adolescent fracture type with three separate fracture planes: one plane oblique in metaphysis, one transverse across physis, one vertical across epiphysis.

1. Mechanism of injury is usually supination-external rotation.
2. May be two-, three-, or four-part fracture.
3. Concern is mainly articular congruity rather than growth remaining (most patients with this fracture are nearing maturity).
4. Treatment
   a. Attempt closed reduction.
   b. If result looks acceptable, confirm with CT scan.
   c. ORIF if there is more than a 2-mm spread or any vertical displacement. Anterolateral incision. Reduce posteromedial fragment first, using a medial incision also if needed.

   F. Salter IV fractures. Reduce and repair if there is any longitudinal displacement or there is a spread greater than 2 mm.

G. Physeal arrest

   1. The **distal tibia** is the third most common site of growth arrest after fracture. This location represents 25% of all physeal bars. It may occur with a Salter II fracture as well as Salter III–V fractures.

   2. Implications

     a. Counsel family on this risk at the time of fracture.

     b. Follow for at least 1 year after injury.

   3. Partial arrest

     a. Calculate potential angulation based on growth remaining.

     b. Guidelines

       (1) 8 mm local growth inhibition = 10-degree deformity will occur if bar forms before age 13½ in boys or age 11½ in girls.

       (2) One cm of growth remains in the distal tibia at age 13 (boys) and after age 11 (girls).

       (3) Refer to growth remaining charts in Chapter 1, Figure 1-20. See also sec. **III.E** in Chapter 1.

   4. Bar resection vs. epiphysiodesis

     a. Epiphysiodesis is simpler and more predictable.

     b. Resection is less crucial in the distal tibia than in other areas of the skeleton because there is less growth in this physis. However, it may be performed if the bar is less than 40% and growth remaining is more than 2 years.

Bibliography

Birch JG. Technique of physeal bar resection. AAOS Instructional Course Lectures 1992. P 445.

Cooperman DR, Spiegel PG, Laros GS. Tibial fractures involving the ankle in children. *J Bone Joint Surg [Am]* 60:1040, 1978.

Dias LS, Giegerich CR. Fractures of the distal tibial epiphysis in adolescence. *J Bone Joint Surg [Am]* 65:438, 1989.Karrholm J, Hansson LI, Selvik G. Longitudinal growth rate of the distal tibia and fibula in children. *Clin Orthop* 191:121, 1984.

Kling TF, Bright RW, Hensinger RN. Distal tibial physeal fractures in children which may require open reduction. *J Bone Joint Surg [Am]* 66:647, 1984.

Schlesinger I, Wedge JH. Percutanoeus reduction and fixation of displaced juvenile Tillaux fractures: A new surgical technique. *J Pediatr Orthop* 13:389, 1993.

Special Procedures

Certain common orthopedic procedures for children are not commonly described. These include techniques for application of traction, administration of regional blocks, and aspiration of major joints. The full descriptions here are a useful guide to medical personnnel.

Chapter Outline

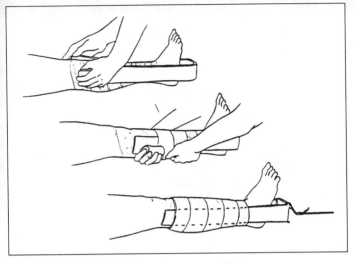

Fig. 6-1. Application of skin traction to lower limb.

I. Skin and skeletal traction

   A. Skin traction. Skin traction is used for conditions requiring moderate traction but not extreme distraction. It is limited by the **shear resistance of skin**, which is approximately **4 lb/limb** in younger children and **5–7 lb/limb** in older children. If these parameters are exceeded, blisters may form. Some indications for skin traction include the following:

      1. Pulling the femoral head down to or past its normal position in developmental dysplasia of the hip up to about age 2–3

      2. Restoring abduction in stiff, adducted hips with Perthes disease

      3. Femur fractures under age 6

         a. As definitive treatment if cast is contraindicated and there is no severe spasticity

         b. As temporary treatment until definitive procedure is performed

      4. For rest to promote resolution of transient synovitis

   B. Skin traction application

      1. Apply benzoin (if desired) followed by a single layer of soft roll. Do not apply the traction strips directly to skin. Application of too much padding would allow traction to slip off when weight is applied.

      2. Place a "U" of adhesive strip to limb, as shown (Fig. 6-1). Be sure to pad the malleoli well. If the traction weight is to approach the limit stated above, distribute the shear by bringing the wrap up to the thigh.

      3. Roll elastic bandage around leg to hold traction strip in place. Do not roll too tightly.

      4. Place spreader in loop of adhesive strip. Make sure the malleoli are free.

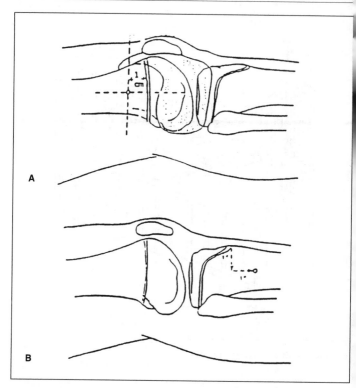

Fig. 6-2. Insertion sites on children for (A) femoral pin and (B) tibial pin.

C. Skeletal traction pin placement

1. Sedate patient, then collect equipment, including Steinmann pin set, hand drill, sterile gloves and towels, lidocaine, syringe with needle, and scalpel.

2. Inject local anesthetic into the entrance and exit areas, being sure to thoroughly numb the periosteum. Femoral nerve block is also an adjunct (see sec. **II.C**).

3. Make small skin incision at the entry site. Use a hemostat to spread the soft tissue down to bone.

4. For a **femoral pin**, enter medially 1 cm above the physis, which is at the adductor tubercle (Fig. 6-2A). For a **tibial pin**, enter laterally 1 cm distal to and posterior to the base of the tibial tubercle (Fig. 6-2B).

5. Have an assistant stabilize the limb with longitudinal traction and counter pressure. Select a pin and insert it into the entry hole. Feel the anterior and posterior edges of the bone by gently "walking" the pin along the cortex. Determine the midpoint and press in the tip of the pin. Adjust the angle of the pin to ensure its exit at the proper position. Maintain pressure.

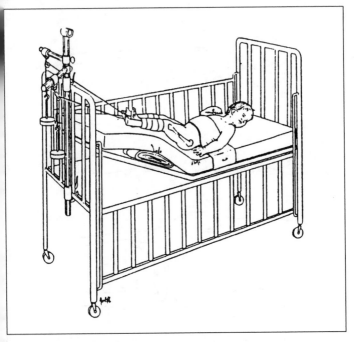

Fig. 6-3. Modified Bryant's traction.

    5. Drill through the bone until the pin tents the skin on the far side.

    6. Make a small incision to allow the pin to exit the skin. Advance pin and place traction bow. Cut any sharp ends off the pin.

D. Traction assembly

    1. Modified Bryant's traction. Use for developmental dysplasia of the hip and hip fractures in infants (Fig. 6-3). Usually flexion of the hip is 30–45 degrees. If a higher angle of flexion is desired, a horizontal bar may be used over the top of the crib.

    2. Split Russell traction. Use in children with hip synovitis or those awaiting treatment of fracture of midshaft of femur (Fig. 6-4). This may be applied as skin or skeletal traction. The hip and knee are flexed 20–30 degrees. The term *split* is used because in the original Russell traction, the same weight was used to provide the vertical as well as the longitudinal traction through a pulley assembly.

    3. Ninety-ninety traction (skeletal traction). The hip and knee are each flexed 90 degrees. Use for definitive treatment of femur fractures in children (Fig. 6-5). It is appropriate for fractures of the proximal, midshaft, or distal femur. Greater supervision is required to obtain

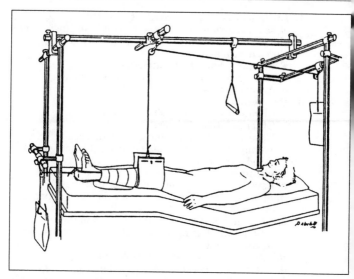

Fig. 6-4. Split Russell traction.

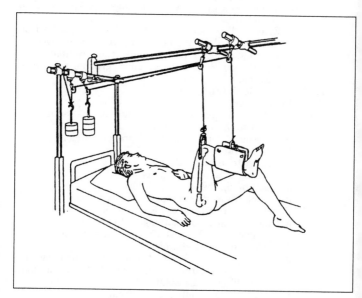

Fig. 6-5. Ninety-ninety (skeletal) traction.

an accurate radiograph with this type of traction than with Bryant's or Russell traction.

II. Regional blocks
A. Intravenous regional anesthesia (Bier block)

1. **Indications.** Upper-extremity fractures requiring closed reduction but not amenable to single-nerve block.
2. **Contraindications**
   a. Fracture above distal humerus
   b. Vascular injury or compartment syndrome
   c. Allergy to local anesthetics
3. **Premedication**
   a. Chloral hydrate, 50–100 mg/kg PO or PR
   b. Other sedative of choice
   c. Have available for administration diazepam (Valium) 1–2 mg IV every 2 minutes as needed for convulsions (incidence <0.5%)
4. **Technique**
   a. Establish IV access in *each* upper extremity.
   b. Apply single- or double-cuff tourniquet on upper arm of injured side.
   c. Exsanguinate by gravity for 1–2 minutes, then inflate cuff. If using double-cuff tourniquet, use most proximal first.
   d. Inflation pressure should be 200 mm Hg.
   e. Inject 0.5% lidocaine 0.6–1.0 ml/kg (3–5 mg/kg).
   f. Reduce fracture; apply splint or cast; confirm with radiograph.
   g. If tourniquet pain occurs, change from proximal to distal cuff.
   h. Release. Tourniquet must be inflated for at least 30 minutes to allow tissue binding of lidocaine. Deflate tourniquet for a few seconds, then reinflate and repeat over 2 minutes to allow gradual release of anesthetic.

B. **Axillary block** (Fig. 6-6)
   1. **Indications**
      a. To provide anesthesia for reduction of fractures of the distal humerus or below.
      b. For wound debridement, closure, or incision
   2. **Contraindications**
      a. Allergy to local anesthetics
      b. Inability to abduct shoulder
      c. Bleeding diathesis
      d. Vascular injury or compartment syndrome
   3. **Premedication to decrease anxiety**
      a. Chloral hydrate 50–100 mg/kg PO or PR.
      b. IV titration with benzodiazepine or narcotic.
   4. Technique of block administration
      a. Draw up anesthetic agent: lidocaine or mepivacaine 5 mg/kg in children, 7 mg/kg in adults (usual adult dose is 40 ml of 1% solution).
      b. IV access and sedation as desired.
      c. Shoulder abduction about 90 degrees.
      d. Palpate axillary artery, pectoralis and latissimus muscles, and humeral head.
      e. Prep and drape axilla.
      f. Puncture skin, and attempt to puncture axillary artery (Fig. 6-6).
      g. Advance needle just through artery with frequent

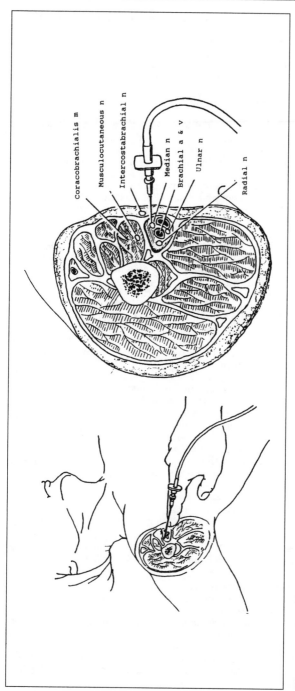

Coracobrachialis m
Musculocutaneous n
Intercostabrachial n
Median n
Brachial a & v
Ulnar n
Radial n

Fig. 6-6. Landmarks for axillary block.

aspiration checks. Inject one-third of anesthetic agent.

h. Slowly withdraw needle to just superficial to artery and inject remainder of agent, 2–3 ml at a time.

i. Apply direct pressure on injection site, and fold extremity across chest to avoid distal runoff of solution.

C. Femoral nerve block

1. Indications

a. Anesthesia of anteromedial thigh or medial aspect of leg or proximal foot (medial border).

b. Minor surgery of anterior thigh

c. Part of multiple lower-extremity block for knee and ankle surgery

d. Relief of postoperative pain in knee

e. Placement and removal of skeletal traction pins

f. Manipulation and reduction of fracture of femur

2. Contraindication: Infection in the groin

3. Technique

a. Draw up anesthetic agent: lidocaine up to 4 mg/kg, or bupivacaine (Marcaine) up to 0.5 mg/kg. (Usual adult dose is 20 ml of 1% lidocaine or 10 ml of 0.5% bupivacaine.)

b. Patient lies supine with thigh on a flat surface.

c. Landmarks (Fig. 6-7)

(1) The femoral nerve is the most lateral structure in the femoral triangle.

(2) Point of entry is one fingerbreadth lateral to the femoral artery below the inguinal ligament.

d. Insertion

(1) Locally infiltrate the point of entry.

(2) Place the middle finger of the nondominant hand on the femoral artery.

(3) Insert the needle one fingerbreadth lateral to the artery cephalad at an angle of 30 degrees.

(4) Once the position of the needle is confirmed, aspirate for blood.

(5) Inject the appropriate volume of local anesthetic if no blood is obtained.

Bibliography

Barnes CL et al. Intravenous regional anesthesia: A safe and cost-effective outpatient anesthetic for upper extremity fracture treatment in children. *J Pediatr Orthop* 11:717, 1991.

III. Injection and aspiration

A. Hip joint aspiration and arthrogram

1. Indications

a. To assess reduction and morphology of the cartilaginous epiphysis.

b. To rule out infection.

2. Hip arthrogram with or without aspiration may be performed via medial (Fig. 6-8), anterior, or lateral (Fig. 6-9)

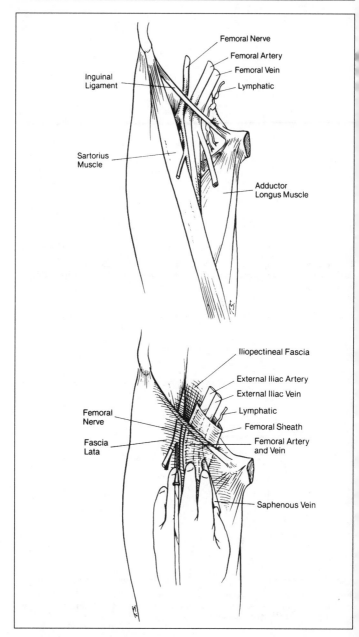

Fig. 6-7. Landmarks for femoral block. Needle insertion is one finger-breadth lateral to femoral artery. (Reproduced with permission from R Prithvi. *Handbook of Regional Anesthesia.* New York: Churchill Livingstone, 1985. P 204.)

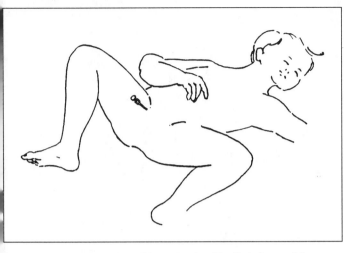

Fig. 6-8. Medial approach for hip aspiration. Needle is inserted just posterior to adductor longus and directed toward anterior superior iliac spine.

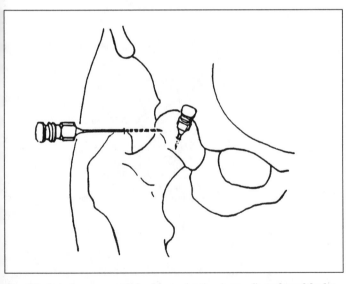

Fig. 6-9. Anterior approach for hip aspiration is two fingerbreadths lateral to femoral artery, below inguinal ligament. Lateral approach is just over the tip of the trochanter.

approach. An arthrogram is usually performed with any aspiration to verify that the needle is within the joint rather than in other tissue spaces. Confirmation of joint entry is important before injecting arthrogram dye to avoid extraarticular contrast material obscuring the field. Confirmation is accomplished by all of the following three methods:

   a. The sensation of the needle popping through the capsule and abutting cartilage (with paradoxical motion on hip rotation)
   b. Radiographic viewing of needle tip
   c. The saline acceptance test

3. **Equipment**
   a. Choice of sedation or anesthesia (or both)
   b. Fluoroscope, fluoroscopy table, shields for physician and patient, or ultrasound
   c. Sterile prep, drape, gloves
   d. Needle, 18- to 20-gauge, 1½ to 3 in. long
   e. Sterile saline (nonbacteriostatic)
   f. Diatrizoate sodium (Renografin-60) for use as contrast medium, diluted to half strength.
   g. Two 10- to 20-cc syringes.
   h. Two IV extension tubes.
   i. Cell count and culture tubes, if needed.

4. **Procedure**
   a. Prep and drape area in a fashion allowing examiner to move the hip during study.
   b. Attach syringes to tubing. Fill one with saline, the other with contrast, and label.
   c. Localize skin entry site and needle direction with fluoroscope.
   d. Advance needle until it is felt to pop through capsule and abut cartilage. There should be paradoxical motion with hip rotation: the needle head should move in the opposite direction of the hip.
   e. Confirm location with x-ray.
   f. Check for mucin string formation on any fluid obtained.
   g. Inject 1–3 ml saline. If it flows easily and much of the fluid can be reaspirated, the needle is in the proper location. If much resistance is encountered, even though needle position is good, it is probably in the femoral head cartilage. If fluid injects easily but does not withdraw, it is probably outside the joint.
   h. If joint fluid is to be analyzed and cultured, do it now (before injecting contrast).
   i. Detach saline-filled syringe and tubing; attach line for contrast medium. Confirm by fluoroscopy during initial injection to detect spill early. Inject just enough dye to outline the joint. If closed reduction is to be performed, minimize capsule distention.
   j. Obtain motion studies and plain x-rays if needed.
   k. If study is done to rule out infection, it is best done in the fluoroscopy suite with sedation rather than in the operating room. This allows adequate time to analyze the joint fluid before deciding on surgery.

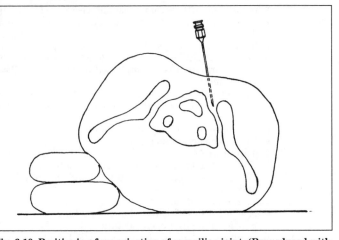

Fig. 6-10. Positioning for aspiration of sacroiliac joint. (Reproduced with permission from RW Hendrix. Simplified aspiration or injection technique for the sacroiliac joint. *J Bone Joint Surg [Am]* 64:1250, 1982.)

B. Sacroiliac joint aspiration
   1. **Indication:** To rule out infection.
   2. **Equipment**
      a. Fluoroscope, table, gowns
      b. Needle (18-gauge, 3 in.)
      c. Preparation and drape towels
      d. Lidocaine
      e. Contrast medium (Renografin-60)
   3. **Technique**
      a. The technique described here takes advantage of the relatively simple plane of the distal third of the joint.
      b. Turn patient prone with unaffected side tilted up 10–30 degrees (Fig. 6-10).
      c. Adjust tilt until caudal third of affected sacroiliac joint is parallel to the beam (Fig. 6-11).
      d. Select needle entry point with fluoroscopy.
      e. Infiltrate skin as necessary.
      f. Insert needle. Check for depth with lateral view as needed.
      g. Aspirate joint; wash with saline as needed.
      h. Confirm joint entry with contrast medium.
      i. Minimize fluoroscopy use because of dose to patient's genitals and surgeon's hands.

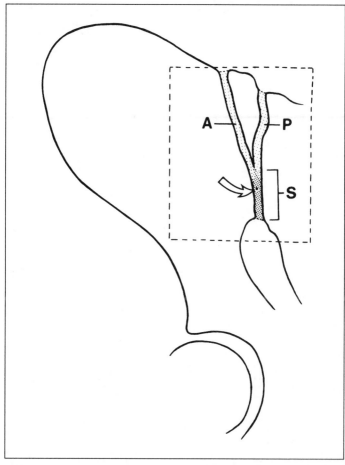

Fig. 6-11. Desired needle placement as seen radiographically. (A = anterior S1 joint; P = posterior S1 joint; S = safe zone.) (Reproduced with permission from RW Hendrix. Simplified aspiration or injection technique for the sacroiliac joint. *J Bone Joint Surg [Am]* 64:1250, 1982.)

Bibliography

Hendrix RW et al. Simplified aspiration or injection technique for the sacroiliac joint. *J Bone Joint Surg [Am]* 64:1249, 1982.

Miskew DB. Aspiration of infected sacroiliac joints. *J Bone Joint Surg [Am]* 64:1071, 1979.

Appendix: Normal Values and Medications

Laboratory values that the pediatric orthopedic surgeon uses frequently are listed in this appendix. Normal laboratory values vary according to age. Medications, including antibiotics, analgesics, and other perioperative drugs, are included with doses and comments.

Pediatric dosages for medication must be calculated based on body weight. Adult doses are given for use in those teenagers and young adults who are fully grown.

When giving agents that affect respiration, the physician should have a plan in place for monitoring and for treatment of any adverse responses.

Table A-1. Normal laboratory values in children
Table A-2. Medications frequently used in pediatric orthopedics
Table A-3. Antibiotics and dosages for children
Table A-4. Latex allergy prevention

Table A-1. Normal laboratory values in children

Age	HCT (%) mean – 2 SD	WBC/mm × 1000 mean ± 2 SD (normal ranges)
Newborn	51 (42)	18.1 (9–30)
6 mos	36 (31)	11.9 (6.0–17.5)
6–24 mos	36 (33)	10.6 (6–17)
2–6 yrs	37 (34)	8.5 (5.0–15.5)
>6 yrs	40 (35)	8.1 (4.5–13.5)

Parameter	Normal values
Sodium	135–145 mg/dl
Potassium	3.5–5.0 mg/dl
Phosphorus	
1–5 yrs	3.5–6.8 mg/dl
>5 yrs	3.0–4.5 mg/dl
Alkaline phosphatase	
Infant	150–400 IU/liter
2–10 yrs	100–300 IU/liter
11–18 yrs (male)	50–375 IU/liter
11–18 yrs (female)	30–300 IU/liter
Erythrocyte sedimentation rate	1–10 mm/hr
Serum creatinine	
Infant	0.2–0.4 mg/dl
Child	0.3–0.7 mg/dl
Adult	0.5–1.0 mg/dl
Glucose	
1 wk–16 yrs	60–105 mg/dl
>16 yrs	70–115 mg/dl
Albumin	
3–4 mos	2.8–5.0 mg/dl
1 yr	3.5–5.0 mg/dl
2 yrs–adult	3.3–5.8 mg/dl
SGPT	
<1 yr	<54 U/liter
>1 yr	1–30 U/liter
SGOT	
<1 yr	25–75 U/liter
>1 yr	0–40 U/liter

Source: MG Greene (ed). *The Harriet Lane Handbook*. St. Louis: Mosby, 1994.

Table A-2. Medications frequently used in pediatric orthopedics

Medication	Dose	Interval	Route	Comments/side effects
Acetaminophen (Tylenol)	65 mg/kg/day (maximum dose)	q4–6h	PO, PR	Hepatotoxicity exacerbates g6PD deficiency.
Albuterol (Proventil, Ventolin)	Usual dose is 10–15 mg/kg/day q4h 2–5 yrs: 0.3 mg/kg/day 6–11 yrs: 2 mg/dose >12 yrs: 2–4 mg/dose Maximum dose: 8 mg PO qid	q8h	PO, inhaler nebulizer	Tachycardia, tremor, nervousness, GI symptoms, HA.
Ascorbic acid (vitamin C)	35–50 mg	qd	PO	
Aspirin (analgesic)	65 mg/kg/day Maximum 3.6 g/day	q4–6h	PO, PR	GI upset, bleeding; do not use for chickenpox or flu-like symptoms. Therapeutic levels: 20–100 mg/liter for use as antipyretic and analgesic; 10–30 mg/dl for use as anti-inflammatory.
Baclofen (Lioresal)	Initial dose 5 mg 2–7 yrs: Increase 5 mg tid q3d to maximum of 10–15 mg tid 7–8 yrs: 20 mg Adult: 20 mg Total daily dose should not exceed 80 mg	tid tid qid	PO	Avoid abrupt withdrawal. Individualize dose.
Beclomethasone (Vanceril, Beclovent)	1–2 inhalations 6–12 yrs maximum: 10 inhalations/24 hrs >12 yrs maximum: 20 inhalations/24 hrs	q6–8h		Not recommended for children <6 yrs old.

Table A-2. (*continued*)

Medication	Dose	Interval	Route	Comments/side effects
Bisacodyl (Dulcolax)	<2 yrs: 5 mg >2 yrs: 10 mg	prn	PR	Effect within 30 min; do not give within 1 hr of antacids or milk.
Calcium carbonate (Os-Cal, Tums)	500 mg–2 g	bid–qid	PO	May cause constipation; take with large glass of water.
Chloral hydrate (sedative or hypnotic)	50–75 mg/kg/dose Maximum dose: 1 g/dose, 2 g/24 hrs	One-time dose only	PO, PR	Contraindicated in hepatic and renal impairment. Caution when using with furosemide and anticoagulants. Use with caution in patients with cardiac disease.
Cimetidine (Tagamet)	Children: 20–40 mg/kg/day Adult: 1.2 g/day	q6h	PO, IV	Use with caution in all patients. May increase serum levels of theophylline, phenytoin, others. Do not use in children <2 yrs; do not administer by IV route.
Codeine	0.5–1.0 mg/kg/dose	q4–6h	PO, IM	
Dantrolene for malignant hyperthermia crisis	1 mg/kg	Repeat until signs and symptoms normalize; up to maximum cumulative dose of 10 mg/kg; then continue at 4–8 mg/kg/24 hrs for 3 days	IV	Contraindicated in active hepatic disease; monitor transaminases.

Drug	Dosage	Interval	Route	Comments
Diazepam (Valium)	Sedative: 0.12–0.8 mg/kg/24 hrs	tid–qid	PO	Not recommended for use in neonates. Do not mix with IV fluids.
	Not for use in children <6 mos 0.04–0.2 mg/kg/dose; maximum dose 0.6 mg/kg within an 8-hr period	q2–4h	IM, IV bolus	
	Anticonvulsant: IV preferable 1 mo–5 yrs: 0.2–0.5 mg/kg/dose; maximum total dose 5 mg	q15–30 min	IV	
	>5 yr: 0.2–0.5 mg/kg/dose; maximum total dose 10 mg	q15–30 min	IV	
	Rate should not exceed 5 mg/min May repeat q15min × 2	q15–30 min	IV	
Diphenhydramine (Benadryl)	Children: 5 mg/kg/day Maximum dose 300 mg/24 hrs	q6h	PO, IV, IM	Contraindicated in infants and neonates, or current MAOI users.
	Adult: 10–50 mg/dose maximum dose 400 mg/24 hrs	q6h–8	PO, IV, IM	
Dimetapp (decongestant, antihistamine)	Adult (PO), children >12 yrs: 4–8 mg	tid–qid	PO	
	For self-medication: 4 mg; maximum 24 mg/24 hrs	q4–6h	PO	
	6–12 yrs: 2–4 mg	tid–qid	PO	
	For self-medication: 2 mg; maximum 12 mg/24 hrs	q4–6h	PO	

Table A-2. (continued)

Medication	Dose	Interval	Route	Comments/side effects
	2–6 yrs: as directed by physician; 1 mg; maximum 6 mg/24 hrs	q4–6h	PO	
	<6 yrs: as directed by physician; 0.5 mg/kg or 15 mg/m^2	tid–qid	PO	
Docusate sodium (laxative; Colace)	<3 yrs: maximum 10–40 mg/24 hrs	qd–qid	PO	
	3–6 yrs: maximum 20–60 mg/24 hrs	qd–qid	PO	
	6–12 yrs: maximum 40–120 mg/24 hrs	qd–qid	PO	
	>12 yrs: maximum 50–240 mg/24 hrs	qd–qid	PO	
Docusate and casanthranol (laxative and stool softener; Peri-Colace)	5–10 ml	qhs	PO	Take with full glass of water.
Fentanyl	0.5–3.0 μg/kg/dose	q1–2h	IV, IM	Give over 3 min for IV dose.
Ferrous sulfate (20% elemental Fe)	For iron-deficiency anemia: 3–6 mg elemental Fe/kg/24 hrs	tid	PO Supplied as: Drops (15 mg Fe/0.6 ml) Syrup (18 mg Fe/5	Do not use in hemolytic disorders. Less GI irritation when given with or after meals. Vitamin C: 200 mg per 30 mg Fe may enhance absorption. May produce constipation, dark stools, nausea, and epigastric

Drug	Dosage	Frequency	Route/Form	Remarks
			ml) Elixir (44 mg Fe/5 ml) Tablets and caps (39, 60, 65, mg Fe/tab)	pain. Antacids may decrease iron absorption. Iron and tetracycline inhibit each other's absorption.
	For prophylaxis: Children: Premature: 2 mg Fe/kg/24 hrs Full term: 1–2 mg Fe/kg/24 hrs Maximum 15 mg/24 hrs	qd–tid	PO	
Folic acid (vitamin supplement)	Adults: 60–100 mg Fe/24 hrs Children: 0.5–1.0 mg/day	qd–bid qd	PO PO	
Furosemide (Lasix)	Adult: 1–3 mg/day Children: 1 mg/kg/dose (may increase by 1 mg/kg/dose)	qd–tid q6–8h prn	PO IV	
Haloperidol (sedative)	Adult: 20–80 mg/dose 0.01–0.1 mg/kg	qd–bid q24h	PO, IV, IM PO	Caution in patients with cardiac disease and in patients with epilepsy.
Hydromorphone (Dilaudid)	1–4 mg Optimum pediatric dosage for analgesia has not been established. As antitussive: children >12 and adults: 1 mg children 6–12: 0.5 mg	q4–6h q3–4h	PO, IV, IM PO	Fewer side effects than morphine sulfate.

Table A-2. (continued)

Medication	Dose	Interval	Route	Comments/side effects
Ibuprofen (Motrin, Advil)	20–40 mg/kg/day (suspension: 100 mg/tsp) (tablets: 200, 300, 400, 600 mg)	q6–8h	PO	GI distress (lessened with milk), rashes, ocular problems. Use caution with aspirin hypersensitivity, or hepatic or renal insufficiency.
Ketamine (hypnotic)	5–7 mg/kg/dose 2–3 mg/kg/dose		IM IV	May cause laryngospasm, hypertension, tachycardia, respiratory depression.
Ketorolac (Toradol)	Children: 1 mg/kg load, 0.5 mg/kg thereafter (not > 30 mg) Adult: 10 mg	q4–6h q6h	IV PO	Do not use parenterally >5 days.
Lidocaine (local anesthetic)	Up to 1 mg/kg for regional block			
Meperidine HCl (Demerol)	Children: 1.0–1.5 mg/kg (maximum 100 mg) Adult: 50–150 mg	q3–4h prn	PO, IM, IV, SC	Contraindicated in cardiac arrhythmia, asthma, increased intracranial pressure. Caution in renal failure.
Methylprednisolone (steroid dose for spinal cord injury)	30 mg/kg bolus then 5.4 mg/kg/hr × 23 hrs	q3–6h prn	PO, IM, IV	
Midazolam (sedative, amnestic; Versed)	0.05–0.15 mg/kg (maximum 5 mg) 1.0 mg/kg	q4h	IV, IM, SC PR	

	Dose	Interval	Route	Notes
Morphine sulfate	0.1–0.3 mg/kg; maximum 15 mg/dose	q4h	IM, SC	IM and IV dose = 6 × PO dose. Naloxone may be used to reverse effects.
	0.1 mg/kg	q2h	IV	
Naloxone (Narcan)	Continuous: 0.025–2.0 mg/kg/hr Single dose: 0.01–0.1 mg/kg/dose Up to maximum 2 mg/dose Repeat q3–5 min	prn	IV, IM	Short acting, may require redose
Naproxen	10 mg/kg/day (suspension: 125 mg/tsp) (tablets: 250, 375 mg)	q12h	PO	
Nystatin (antifungal, topical)	Infants: 1 ml; Children and adults: 4–6 ml; swish and swallow	q6h	PO	May produce diarrea and GI symptoms.
Ondansetron (Zofran)	4 yrs–adult: 0.15 mg/kg/dose	May repeat 1–3 times q4h	IV	
Oxycodone	Children: 0.05–0.15 mg/kg/dose Adult: 5 mg	q6h	PO	Abuse potential; urinary retention.
Paraldehyde (sedative, hypnotic)	Anticonvulsant: 0.3 ml/kg/dose in 1:1 dilution with cottonseed or olive oil (PR) Sedative: 0.15 ml/kg/dose (diluted in milk or fruit juice)		IM, PO, PR	Avoid plastic equipment. Contraindicated in hepatic or pulmonary disease.
Paregoric (analgesic)	0.25–0.5 ml/kg/dose	qd–q6h	PO	

Table A-2. *(continued)*

Medication	Dose	Interval	Route	Comments/side effects
Prochlorperazine (antiemetic; Compazine)	0.4 mg/kg/day	q6–8h	PO, PR	Child >2 yrs or >10 kg only.
	0.1–0.15 mg/kg (single dose)		IM	
Promethazine (Phenergan)	0.25–0.50 mg/kg/dose	q4–6h prn	IM, PR	
Ranitidine (Zantac)	2–4 mg/kg/day	q12h	PO	
	1–2 mg/kg/day	q6–8h	IV	
	Child weighing 15–40 kg: 100–200 mg	q6–8h	PO	CNS disturbances are common in children. Injection not recommended for children <14 yrs.
Trimethobenzamide (antiemetic; Tigan)	PR (not for use in neonates)			
	<15 kg: 100 mg	tid–qid	PR	
	>15 kg: 100–200 mg	tid–qid	IM	

Table A-3. Antibiotics and dosages for children

Drug	Dose	Interval	Route	How supplied	Comments
Amikacin	15 mg/kg/day maximum: 1.5 g/24 hrs	q8h	IV, IM	Injection: 50, 250 mg/ml	Monitor levels: Peak 20–30 mg/liter, trough 5–10 mg/liter. Adjust dose with renal impairment. Ototoxic effects with lasix.
Amoxicillin	Child: 20–40 mg/kg/day Adult: 250–500 mg/dose	q8h	PO	Drops: 50 mg/ml; suspension: 125, 250 mg/5 ml Caps: 250, 500 mg; chewable: 125, 250 mg	Less GI irritation than ampicillin.
Amoxicillin and clavulanic acid (Augmentin)	Child: 20–40 mg/kg/day	q8h	PO	Suspension: 125, 250 mg/5 ml; tablets: 250–500 mg; chewable: 125, 250 mg	Used with *H. influenzae*, *Staphylococcus aureus*, beta-lactamase producers.
Ampicillin	50–100 mg/kg/day	q6h	PO, IM, IV	Drops: 100 mg/ml; suspension: 125, 250, 500 mg/5 ml	Maximum oral dose 2–4 g/day; may cause nephritis.
Carbenicillin	400–500 mg/kg/day maximum: 40 g/24 hrs	q4h–q6h	IV (cut dose to one-half)		Use with caution in renal impairment or penicillin allergy.

Table A-3. (continued)

Drug	Dose	Interval	Route	How supplied	Comments
Cefaclor (Ceclor)	40 mg/kg/day maximum: 2 g/24 hrs	q8h	PO		Use with caution in renal impairment or penicillin allergy.
Cefadroxil (Duricef, Ultracef)	Infant and child: 30 mg/kg/day Adult: 1–2 g/day	q12h q12h	PO PO		Use with caution in renal impairment or penicillin allergy.
Cefamandole (Mandol)	Children: 50–150 mg/kg/day Adult: 4–12 g/day	q4–6h q4–8h	IM, IV IM, IV		Use with caution in renal impairment or penicillin allergy.
Cefazolin (Ancef, Kefzol)	Infant and child: 25–100 mg/kg/day	q6-8h	IM, IV		Use with caution in renal failure or penicillin allergy.
Cefoperazone (Cefobid)	Children: 100–200 mg/kg/day Adult: 2–4 g/day	q12h q12h	IM, IV IM, IV		Use with caution in renal failure or penicillin allergy.
Cefotaxime (Claforan)	Infant and child: 50–200 mg/kg/day Adult (>50 kg): 2–12 g/day	q4–6h q4–12h	IM, IV IM, IV		Use with caution in renal failure or penicillin allergy.
Cefoxitin (Mefoxin)	Infant and child: 80–160 mg/kg/day Adult: 4–12 g/day	q4–6h q6–8h	IM, IV IM, IV		Use with caution in renal failure or penicillin allergy. (contains 2.3 Na/g).

Drug	Dose	Interval	Route	Forms	Comments
Ceftazidime (Fortaz, Ceptaz)	Infant and child: 90–150 mg/kg/day	q8h	IM, IV		Use with caution in renal failure or penicillin allergy (contains 2.3 Na/g).
	Adult: 2–6 g/day	q8–12h	IM, IV		
Ceftizoxime (Cefizox)	Infant and child: 150–200 mg/kg/day	q6–8h	IM, IV		Use with caution in renal failure or penicillin allergy.
	Adult: 2–12 g/day	q8–12h	IM, IV		
Ceftriaxone (Rocephin)	Infant and child: 50–75 mg/kg/day	q12–24h	IM, IV		Use with caution in renal impairment or penicillin allergy.
	Adult: 1–4 g/day	q12h	IM, IV		
Cefuroxime (Zinacef, Kefurox)	Infant and child: 50–100 mg/kg/day	q6–8h	IM, IV		Use with caution in renal impairment or penicillin allergy.
	Adult: 2.25–9 g/day	q6–8h	IM, IV		
Cephalexin (Keflex)	Infant and child: 25–50 mg/kg/day	q6–12h	PO	Drops: 100 mg/ml; suspension: 125, 250 mg/5 ml; tablets: 1,000 mg; capsules: 250, 500 mg	Use with caution in renal insufficiency.
	Adult: 1–4 g/day	q6–12h	PO		
Cephalothin (Keflin)	Child: 80–160 mg/kg/day	q4–6h	IV, IM (deep)		
	Adult: 2–12 g/day	q4–6h	IM, IV		

Table A-3. (continued)

Drug	Dose	Interval	Route	How supplied	Comments
Chloramphenicol	Children and adults: 50–100 mg/kg/day maximum: 4 g/24 hrs	q6h	PO, IV		Monitor levels in infants.
Ciprofloxacin (Cipro)	250–750 mg 200–400 mg	bid q12h	PO IV		Not recommended for children <16 yrs; monitor if renal impairment.
Clindamycin (Cleocin)	Children: 10–25 mg/kg/day 10–40 mg/kg/day Adult: 600–1800 mg/day 600–3600 mg/day	q6–8h q6–8h q6–8h q6–8h	PO IM, IV PO IV	Caps: 75, 150, 300 mg Suspension: 75 mg/5 ml	May cause pseudomembranous enterocolitis; caution in hepatic or renal insufficiency.
Cloxacillin (Tegopen)	Children: 50–100 mg/day Adult: 250–1,000 mg/dose Maximum: 4 g/24 hrs	qid qid	PO PO	Caps: 250, 500 mg Sol: 125 mg/5 ml	Give on empty stomach.
Dicloxacillin (Dynapen)	Child (<40 kg): 25 mg/kg/day Adult: 1–2 g/day Maximum: 4 g/24 hrs	2 hrs after meals qid	PO PO		

Drug	Dosage	Frequency	Route	Preparations	Notes
Doxycycline (Vibramycin)	< 45 kg: 5 mg/kg for 1 day to maximum of 200 mg/24 hrs > 45 kg: 200 mg/24 hrs for 1 day	q12h q12h	PO, IV	Capsules/tablets: 50, 100 mg; suspensions: 25 mg/5 ml	Not for children <8 yrs. Caution in hepatic and renal disease. Avoid direct sunlight.
Erythromycin	Children: 30–50 mg/kg/day Maximum: 2 g/24 hrs Adult: 1–4 g/day Maximum: 4 g/24 hrs	q6–8h q6h	PO, IV PO, IV		Multiple GI discomfort; give after meals; caution with liver disease. Avoid IM route.
Ethambutol (Myambutol)	15–25 mg/kg/day	qd	PO		Not for children <12 yrs. Give with food. Adjust dose with renal failure.
Gentamicin	Children: 6.0–7.5 mg/kg/day Maximum: 300 mg/24 hrs Adult: 3–5 mg/kg/day	q8h q8h	IV, IM IV, IM		Monitor levels: peak 6–10 mg/liter; trough 2 mg/liter. Monitor renal status; watch for ototoxicity.
Methicillin (Staphcillin)	Children: 100–400 mg/kg/day Adult: 4–12 g/day Maximum: 12 g/24 hrs	q4–6h q4–6h	IM, IV IM, IV		See product guidelines for neonatal dosage.

Table A-3. (continued)

Drug	Dose	Interval	Route	How supplied	Comments
Metronidazole (Flagyl)	Children and adults: Load with 15 mg/kg dose beginning 48 hrs after loading dose. Then 7.5 mg/kg/	q6–12h	IV IV, PO		Do not ingest alcohol for 24 hrs after dose. Except for amebiasis, safe use of Metronidazole in children <12 yrs has not been established.
Oxacillin	Children: 50–100 mg/kg/day Adult: 2–4 g/day	q6h q6h	PO		
Penicillin G (potassium or sodium)	Children: 100,000–300,000 units/ kg/day 25–50 mg/kg Adult: 1.2–24.0 million units/day	q4–6h q6 q4–6h	PO IV, IM PO IV, IM		Probenecid may prolong availability Penicillin G must be taken 1–2 hrs before or 2 hrs after meals. 1 mg = 1,600 units
Penicillin G (Benzathine)	1–2 g Children: 50,000 U/day Maximum: 2.4 million units Adult: 1.2 million units	q6h One dose	PO IM		Provides sustained levels for 2–4 wks
Penicillin G (Procaine)	Children: 25,000–50,000 U/kg/day	q12–24h	IM		Provides sustained levels for 2–4 days

Drug	Dose	Frequency	Route	Comments
Penicillin V potassium	Adult: 600,000–1 million units/day Children: 25–50 mg/kg/day	q6h	PO	Must be taken 1 hr before or 2 hrs after meals.
Rifampin	Adult: 1–2 g/day	q6h	PO	Colors secretions red. Give 1 hr before or 5 hrs after meals. Caution in liver disease.
	Children > 1 mo: 20 mg/kg/dose Maximum: 600 mg/dose for 2 days if meningitis prophylaxis Maximum: 600 mg/24 hrs for 4 days if *H. influenzae*	q12h (meningitis) q24h (TB) qd	PO, IV	
Tetracycline HCl	Older child: 25–50 mg/kg/day Adult: 1–2 g/day	q6h	PO	Not for children <8 yrs or in pregnancy. Give 1 hr before or 2 hrs after meals. Do not give with dairy products.
Ticarcillin (Ticar)	200–300 mg/kg/day Maximum: 24–30 g/24 hrs	q4–6h	IM, IV	Contains sodium—each g = 5.2–6.5 mEq Na^+.

Table A-3. (*continued*)

Drug	Dose	Interval	Route	How supplied	Comments
Tobramycin	Children: 6.0–7.5 mg/kg/day	q8h	IV, IM		Check levels: peak 6–10 mg/liter; trough <2 mg/liter.
	Adult: 3–5 mg/kg/day				
Vancomycin	Children: 10 mg/kg/dose	q8h	IV		Benadryl can reverse red man syndrome.
	Adult: 2 g/day	q6–12h			

Bibliography

Jackson MA, Nelson JD. Management of bone and joint infections in pediatric patients. *J Pediatr Orthop* 2:313, 1982.

Johns Hopkins Pharmacy Formulary, 1996.

Johnson KD. *The Harriet Lane Handbook.* St. Louis: Mosby-Year Book, 1993.

Physician's Desk Reference. Oradell, NJ: Medical Economics, 1993.

Medical Letter Handbook of Antimicrobial Therapy. New York: Medical Letter, 1994.

AHFS Drug Information. Bethesda, MD: American Hospital Formulary Service, 1995.

Table A-4. Latex allergy prevention

Etiology: Multiple exposures, genetic predisposition (?)
Conditions that place patients at risk:
    Myelodysplasia
    Exstrophy
    Cerebral palsy with shunt
    Other congenital urologic anomalies
Management: Avoid exposure to latex. Treat acute episodes with
    epinephrine, bronchodilators, steroids, and volume.

Latex-containing item	Latex-free item
Gloves: Eudermic, Ultraderm, Micro-Touch, Bio Gel D, Neutralon, Perry Derma-Guard, Safeskin, Pristine, Sensi-Derm, Neutraderm, Brown Milled, Baxter Exam Gloves	Safe gloves: Tactylon, Neolon, Dermaprene, Elastyren, vinyl exam gloves
Cloth tape	3M tapes (Microfoam/Micropore)
Coban Dressings	Silktape
	Steri-drapes (3M)
Band-Aids	Dermaclear/dermacil tape (Johnson & Johnson)
	Nelcor oximeter probes
	Steri-strips (3M), Tegaderm (3M)
Red rubber urinary catheters	Catheters: ureteral, suction, silastic, Foley catheters, (Argyle, Bard, Surgicath, Mentor) Ureteral catheter (Surgicath), Vessiloops (Devon Industries), silicone Foley catheters (Sherwood)
Red rubber endotracheal tubes	Plastic oral airways
	Standard endotracheal tubes (Portex, Mallinkrodt)
Red rubber nasopharyngeal airways (Rusch)	Portex nasal airways
	Ear tubes (Richard, Xomed)
Penrose drains	Jackson-Pratt drains, Hemovac drains (latex inside)
Dental dams	
BP cuff and attached tubing	
Tourniquets	
IV tubing injection ports	Xeroform (Sherwood Medical)
Buretrol latex diaphragm	Salem sump tubes
Nondisposable temperature probes	
Black anesthesia masks	
Ventilator bellows*	
Fresh gas flow anesthesia machine tubing	
Nuk nipples and some other feeding nipples and pacifiers	
Medication vial stoppers	

*Not thought to be a risk with usual use.

Bibliography

Dormans JP. Intraoperative anaphylaxis due to exposure to latex in children. *J Bone Joing Surg [Am]* 76:1688, 1994.

Emans JB. Current concepts review: Allergy to latex in patients who have myelodysplasia. Relevance for the orthopedic surgeon. *J Bone Joint Surg [Am]* 74:1103, 1992.

Index